VISION, PERCEPTION and COGNITION

A Manual for the Evaluation and Treatment of the Neurologically Impaired Adult

Third Edition

VISION, PERCEPTION and COGNITION

A Manual for the Evaluation and Treatment of the Neurologically Impaired Adult

Third Edition

Barbara Zoltan, MA, OTR

Previously published under the title:
Perceptual Dysfunction in the Adult Stroke Patient:
A Manual for Evaluation and Treatment
by Ellen Siev and Brenda Freishtat
and under the title
The Adult Stroke Patient:
A Manual for Evaluation and Treatment of Perceptual and Cognitive Dysfunction
Revised Second Edition
by Barbara Zoltan, Ellen Siev, and Brenda Freishtat

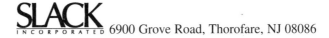 6900 Grove Road, Thorofare, NJ 08086

Zoltan, Barbara.
Vision, perception, and cognition: a manual for the evaluation and treatment of the neurologically impaired adult/Barbara Zoltan. -- 3rd ed.
    p. cm.
"Previously published under the title: Perceptual and cognitive dysfunction in the adult stroke patient: a manual for evalution and treatment by Ellen Siev, Brenda Freishtat, and Barbara Zoltan."
Includes bibliographical references and index.
ISBN 1-55642-265-2 (alk. paper)
    1. Cerebrovascular disease--Patients--Rehabilitation. 2. Perception, Disorders of. 3. Cognition disorders. 4. Visual agnosia. I. Siev, Ellen. Perceptual and cognitive dysfunction in the adult stroke patient. II. Title.
    [DNLM: 1. Cerebrovascular Disorders--rehabilitation. 2. Brain Injuries--rehabilitation. 3. Vision Disorders--diagnosis. 4. Vision Disorders--therapy. 5. Cognition Disorders--diagnosis. 6. Cognition Disorders--therapy. WL 355 Z86v 1996]
    RC388.5.Z65 1996
    616.8'103--dc20
    DNLM/DLC
    for Library of Congress   96-24230
                                                                                           CIP

Printed in the United States of America.

Published by: SLACK Incorporated
                  6900 Grove Road
                  Thorofare, NJ 08086 USA
                  Telephone: 856-848-1000
                  Fax: 856-853-5991
                  www.slackbooks.com

    Last digit is print number: 10

Dedication

This book is dedicated to Les, Adam and Scott
for their love, patience and understanding.

Contents

Acknowledgments

For time and ideas:
Mary Warren, MS, OTR
Joan P. Toglia, MA, OTR
Karin Bonfils, OTR
&
Rick Parente, PhD

For manuscript preparation:
Dianne Wall

About the Author

Barbara Zoltan, MA, OTR, is a consultant in private practice in Northern California. She obtained her BS in Occupational Therapy from Tufts University and her master's degree from the University of Southern California. She holds certifications in both sensory integration and neurodevelopmental treatment and serves on the editorial boards of the *Journal of Head Trauma Rehabilitation* and *Occupational Therapy in Health Care*. Her 20 years of experience specializing in neurological rehabilitation has included a broad range of research, teaching, administrative and clinical practice. She has published over 20 articles, chapters and books related to the rehabilitation of the adult with neurological deficits.

Introduction

More than half a million cerebral vascular accidents (C.V.A.) occur annually in the United States, and at any given time, there are 2 million people who have survived a C.V.A.[1-3] Of those surviving the initial insult, 50 percent will live another five years and 75 percent will be rehabilitated to some degree of independence. Of these new patients, 60 to 70 percent can expect to become ambulatory, although significant functional return of the affected upper extremity is expected in only 30 to 40 percent. There are over 422,000 new cases of traumatic brain injury (T.B.I.) each year.[1,4] At any given time, approximately 926,000 people sustain deficits to the extent that they require services.[4]

Until recently, rehabilitation focused on restoration of motion and compensation for lost functional skills. Visual, perceptual and cognitive deficits, noted for many years to exist as a result of cerebral vascular accidents or T.B.I., have only recently been acknowledged as a cause of continued confusion and lack of rehabilitation progress in many patients even though motor skills have returned. As many as two thirds of all T.B.I. patients experience some type of cognitive loss.[5] Recent research has clearly shown a significant relationship between visual, perceptual and/or cognitive loss and functional abilities.[5-8]

Despite the prevalence of C.V.A and T.B.I. patients, the formulation of definitive evaluation and treatment techniques remains incomplete at best. This manual was completed after extensive research and clinical experience and is intended to reflect the current state of the art in the evaluation and treatment of visual, perceptual and cognitive processing deficits for the adult with neurological impairment. It is intended to be a resource book, and as such the material has been documented as closely as possible for future referencing. Generally, theoretical information is included as well as specific theoretical information pertaining to each sub-component skill. The application of this information to practice through specific frames of reference is also provided. Finally, specific evaluation and treatment techniques based on this theoretical information are outlined.

It is my goal that this manual be useful for both the student and the experienced clinician. It is also my hope that it will foster good clinical reasoning skills and stimulate future research.

Barbara Zoltan, MA, OTR

References

1. Allen CK. Treatment plans in cognitive rehabilitation. *Occup Ther Pract.* 1989;1(1):1-8.

2. Joe BE. Accelerating stroke rehab. *OT Week*. 1995;9(42):14-15.

3. McCollough NC III, Sarniento A. Functional prognosis of the hemiplegic. *J Florida Med Assoc*. 1970;57:31-34.

4. Vogenthaler DR. Rehabilitation after closed head injury: A primer. *J Rehab*. Oct/Nov/Dec 1987.

5. Kaplan CP and Corrigan JD. The relationship between cognition and functional independence in adults with traumatic brain injury. *Arch Phys Med Rehabil*. June 1994;75:643-647.

6. Edmans JA and Lincoln NB. The frequency of perceptual deficits after stroke. *Clinical Rehab*. 1987;1:273-281.

7. Rubio KB and Van Deusen J. Relation of perceptual and body image dysfunction to activities of daily living of persons after stroke. *Amer J of Occup Ther*. 1995;49(6):551-559.

8. Titus MLD, Gall NG, Yerxa EJ, Roberson TA and Mack W. Correlation of perceptual performance and activities of daily living in stroke patients. *Amer J Occup Ther*. 1991;45(5):410-417.

CHAPTER 1

Theoretical Basis for Evaluation and Treatment

Occupational therapy, as with any scientific profession, requires a conceptual foundation with underlying assumptions to guide practice decisions. These theoretical concepts are generally structured into models. Portions of these models, which are methodological in emphasis, form a frame of reference.[1] The frame of reference is the mechanism which links theory to practice.[2] Occupational therapy contains many frames of reference depending on the patient population or specific area of focus. Although these frames of reference have been effective to some degree, it is only recently that the profession has begun to relate them to an overall theoretical basis for occupational therapy practice.

Every occupational therapist would agree that the profession is based on the concept of human occupation. Referrals are made because of the patient's inability to perform daily life tasks, which prevents independence and return to previous social roles. Not all occupational therapists however, would agree on how to evaluate and treat these inabilities. Many therapists advocate for the need to evaluate component skills such as attention, memory or strength as a means to help clarify the cause of occupational performance deficits and assist in treatment planning.[3] Assumptions are made based on established research, about the correlation of specific component deficits to the patient's problems with occupational performance.[4] This method of evaluating and testing component skills has recently come into question. Some therapists believe this approach to be reductionistic and recommend a more holistic focus of evaluation and treatment.[5-7] It is felt that "...while a certain causal relationship does exist whereby improvement in the microlevel of cognitive components of performance may result in improved occupational performance in real life, a large variance in actual performance abilities cannot be explained by looking at or treating the micro-level alone."[6] These therapists believe that occupational performance should be the primary focus of occupational therapy assessment and treatment.[3]

As with any controversy, critical thinking or questioning often results in an improved perspective. This perspective leads to the incorporation of ideas from many sides and the formation of a solution which is useful and beneficial to all practitioners. Catherine Trombly, for example, answers to the labeling of component skills evaluation as "reductionistic" as follows.

If a hierarchical theory of occupational functioning that includes abilities and capacities is accepted, then the assessment process should include these levels....the assessment should not be considered a reductionistic one, but rather an augmentative one that relates and extends each level toward occupational functioning.[8]

Abreu et al support the need for multiple level evaluation and treatment in their description of the new functional treatment. They encourage therapists to evaluate the patient at both the micro and macro levels of occupational functioning so that abilities and skills can be reliably monitored at both levels.[5] Ben-Yishay and Diller describe cognitive difficulties as "layered and coexistent."[9,10] They also recommend a systematic, multi-model approach to cognitive rehabilitation. Farrell et al, believe the effective remediation of visuo-motor deficits requires a systematic approach within a hierarchical framework.

Research which clarifies the relationship between components and higher level skills, as well as the minimal abilities required to accomplish activities that compose tasks of particular roles, is needed.[8] Extensive tool development is also needed for the evaluation of role performance, occupational performance and performance components. Measures which evaluate the thinking demands of day to day living are just recently being developed. The processes by which patients solve problems are being analyzed in addition to the scores themselves.[11]

In summary, the theoretical basis for evaluation and treatment need not include one level of focus to the exclusion of another. Evaluation and treatment which focus on deficits of components of function thought to be prerequisites of occupational performance have been termed *bottom-up assessment*.[8] Examining role competence, the tasks which define these roles and what the patient can and cannot do, is termed *top-down assessment*.[8] The combination of both top-down and bottom-up assessment and treatment of occupational functioning will give the clearest picture of the patient's overall functioning at all levels. The therapist should choose a combination of assessments and treatments to provide the most complete picture of the patient in the least amount of time.[1] In order to make these decisions, the therapist must understand the underlying concepts and have a framework for organizing and interpreting information.

The theoretical basis for the treatment of visual, perceptual and cognitive deficits has traditionally been divided into two categories, *adaptive* and *remedial*.[12] There are many factors which may dictate whether the remedial or adaptive approach or a combination of the two approaches is utilized. The current state of the health care system in general and trend of shorter hospital stays, for example, may necessitate the use of an adaptive approach. Many believe, however, that by combining both schools of thought we can best meet the needs of our patients.[8,12,13]

One factor which must be considered in making a choice between a remedial or adaptive approach is the patient's ability to learn.[14] In order to utilize the remedial approach, the patient must have some learning capacity.[15] The therapist must identify what modes of input the patient can process most easily, what approaches to tasks are still available to the patient, and what tasks are still meaningful to the patient.[15]

A variety of frames of reference for treatment have been operationalized and fall within either a remedial or adaptive conceptual base. The underlying assumptions of this conceptual base are subsequently described in this chapter. In addition, the frames of reference which are most widely utilized by occupational therapists are reviewed. The theoretical information presented is meant as an overview and the reader is encouraged to seek out additional references and certification as needed. The information presented in this chapter is then applied and integrated into later portions of the book which provide specific evaluation and treatment techniques.

Remedial Approach

The remedial approach, at times termed the restorative approach, focuses on the impairment underlying the disability.[8,11,12,16,17] It utilizes repeated drills and exercises which are aimed at specific cognitive processes in an attempt to promote new neural connections and recovery of function.[8,12,18] It is assumed that the brain can repair itself by reestablishing synaptic connections or growing new ones.[19] It is also assumed with a remedial approach, that occupational performance is composed of subcomponents which can be "...remediated by a building block approach that emphasizes improvement of hierarchical elements/subcomponents to allow the structure of occupational performance to be reconstructed."[17] The goal of the remedial approach is to increase and improve the patient's ability to process and use incoming information so as to allow increased function in everyday life.[9,13] Remedial treatment is a *bottom up approach* which assumes the patient will be able to generalize to activities of daily living.[8] It is assumed that "...if one trains to remediate an impaired core area of cognitive function, the individual will be able to resume competent functioning in those daily life situations that involve these core functions."[9] Some research has shown, however, that a restorative approach to some subcomponent skills has had a limited direct impact on the enhancement of functional activities.[9,20] Some examples of remedial approaches are Sensory Integrative, Affolter and Neurodevelopmental.

Adaptive Approach

The adaptive approach is a *top down approach* which promotes adaptation of and to the environment to capitalize on the patient's abilities. Adaptive approaches provide training in actual occupational behaviors and are traditionally used when restoration is unlikely.[8,19] Adaptive approaches facilitate improved function through compensation. Compensation is any practical environmental adjustment "...made to make up for performance deficits" (eg, adaptive equipment, assistance from a caregiver or training procedures that are activity or situation specific).[21]

Compensation can be *external*, which is assistance provided by outside sources, or *situational*, which is a technique utilized by the patient so he does not depend on others.[22] In order to utilize situational compensation techniques, the patient must have at least some awareness of existing deficits. This awareness may cause the patient to be frustrated with his performance, however, it will help motivate him to learn new strategies.[20] Compensatory behaviors are most successful when they are overlearned to the point of automatic.[17] In addition, compensation strategies should be practiced in a variety of different environments.[6] The choice and design of activity or environmental compensations is based on the therapist's understanding of disability and activity analysis.[21] Some examples of adaptive approaches are Functional, Occupational Performance, and Dynamic Interactional Approach.

Frames of Reference Utilizing a Remedial Conceptual Base

Bottom-Up Approaches

Sensory Integration

The sensory integrative approach is used most often by occupational therapists when treating perceptual, cognitive, and behavioral problems in children. The sensory integrative model for treatment is based on neurophysiological and developmental principles, and can be defined as the organization of sensation for use by the individual.[23] Integration converts our initial sensations into meaningful perceptions. Spatial organization, for example, is based on the integration of an assortment of visual, auditory, and kinesthetic cues.[23] Sensory integration is the processing and organizing function of the brain and the manner in which disparate sensations are related to each other.[24] Once sensations are related to each other, they develop significance, which guides an adaptive response which is either motor or cognitive. Sensory integration, through environmental interaction, "...contributes to the development of perception, orientation in space, coordination, skilled movement and primary cognitive processes."[24] If sensory integration is impaired, the resulting perceptions of an individual are distorted. How well an individual processes information from visual, proprioceptive, tactile and auditory systems and "...how well inputs from one sensory channel to another are related, determine that person's ability to interact appropriately and effectively with his environment."[25] Sensory motor integration can occur at all levels of the central nervous system, extending from the spinal cord to the cerebral cortex.[23]

Sensory integration occurs during an adaptive response.[26] The adaptive response is both goal directed and purposeful. During sensory integrative therapy, the therapist provides and controls sensory input, especially the input from the vestibular system, muscles, joints, and skin. This controlled sensory stimulation is then followed by an adaptive response by the patient, which will integrate those sensations provided and controlled by the therapist. The emphasis of sensory integrative therapy is on the integration of vestibular, proprioceptive and tactile input, not just on the motor response.[27]

In recent years, a new conceptual focus of sensory integration theory has been described which incorporates concepts from an occupational behavior framework. Fisher and Murray hypothesize "...that through a spiral process of self-actualization, sensory integration and the corresponding adaptive behaviors lead to organized and appropriate occupational behavior."[27] As a child grows and develops control over the environment, interaction becomes more meaningful and satisfying.[27]

Although originally developed for use with children, there is increased interest on the part of occupational therapists in the use of sensory integrative therapy with brain-damaged adults. The use of sensory integrative therapy with brain-damaged adults, however, remains controversial. Jongbloed, Collins and Jones state that many professionals who provide perceptual training to brain-damaged adults have found an inability of many patients to organize and process information from different sensory channels, and do not relate inputs from one channel to another in responding to their environment.[25] In other words, these patients exhibit poor sensory integrative functioning. Documentation of this dysfunction in adult T.B.I. or C.V.A. patients has increased.[28,29]

Fisher and Murray, however, believe that the diagnosis of sensory integrative dysfunction requires that evidence of the problem not be attributable to either peripheral or cortical central nervous system dysfunction.[27] These authors state that it is unlikely that an older person with adult onset learning would have sensory integrative problems unless that individual had sensory integration problems as a child.[27] Abreu and Toglia also question the use of techniques which were designed for the young developing brain and believe that techniques which emphasize acquiring new skills may not be easily applied to a brain that has already acquired such skills.[6]

Justification for the use of sensory integration therapy with the adult C.V.A. and T.B.I. patient is based on concepts and documented studies in several related areas: aging, the effect of environment on central nervous system functioning, and brain plasticity. The majority of the stroke population are 60 years old or older.[30] One study indicated that 81 percent of the stroke population were 65 to 74 years old and that 92.5 percent were between 75 and 84.[31] It is documented that the well, elderly individual experiences changes in all sensory systems, perception, and intellectual functioning. These changes are described in detail in *The Relationship of Age to Visual, Perceptual and Cognitive Evaluation and Treatment* in Chapter 11.

The most relevant changes relative to the elderly (well or brain-damaged) and the application of sensory integration are those of the primary sensory systems and the vestibular system. Recent research indicates that there is a decrease in the quantity and diameter of vestibular nerves in the elderly, as well as decreased vestibular reflexes.[32] Age related changes in the sensory components of the central nervous system can result in impaired processing of both the internal and the external environments.[33] Memory loss, one of the most devastating impairments experienced by the elderly, has been linked with modality specific sensory memory.[33] Ordy et al state, "...convergent polysensory information processing in multimodal sensory integration within the cerebral cortex and limbic system may play a critical role in the short-term memory impairment of the elderly."[33]

It is well documented that elderly patients lose the ability to adapt effectively to the environment, and that autonomic nervous system changes decrease their ability to make adaptive responses. In addition, the elderly experience increasing sensory isolation, which can in turn lead to functional and structural changes in vital sensory links that guide and facilitate adaptation and behavior.[33]

Table 1-1 summarizes normal sensory integrative functioning and that of the elderly individual. The sensory integrative dysfunction present in the elderly is similar to that in the learning disabled child. It can be hypothesized that some sensory integrative techniques successfully utilized with the learning disabled child can also be effective with the well or brain-damaged elderly with similar dysfunction.

The second factor to consider when relating sensory integration and the adult patient is the environment. As previously noted, a major theoretical construct of sensory integration is the necessity for sensory stimulation from the environment for normal functioning. The need for environmental stimulation is emphasized when one considers the results of environmental deprivation. Studies of institutionalized geriatric patients indicated a decrease in the quality of

TABLE 1-1. SUMMARY OF NORMAL SENSORY INTEGRATIVE FUNCTION AND THAT OF THE ELDERLY INDIVIDUAL

Normal	Elderly (Well or Brain Damaged)
Sensory stimulation from the environment	Sensory stimulation from the environment
↓	↓
Normal sensory registration and processing	Abnormal sensory registration and processing due to impaired primary sensory systems (ie, visual, auditory, tactile, olfactory, and gustatory)
↓	↓
Normal sensory integration and interpretation	Abnormal sensory integration and interpretation due to impaired primary sensory systems and impaired autonomic, proprioceptive, and vestibular systems
↓	↓
Appropriate functional adaptive response	Poor and inappropriate adaptive response due to impaired primary sensory systems, impaired autonomic, proprioceptive, and vestibular systems and age or disability related mobility impairment.

verbalization, difficulties in directed thinking and concentration, drifting of thought, disorientation in time, and complaints of restlessness.[34]

A sensory deprivation study of normal adults indicated that the subjects exhibited a general disorganization of brain function similar to that produced by anoxia or brain tumors.[35]

Although the patient who has sustained a C.V.A. is not in a sensory-deprived environment, the limitations caused by the C.V.A. result in the same situation as that of a sensory-deprived environment. When an individual suffers a C.V.A. or T.B.I. that individual's mobility will be limited. This limitation in mobility in turn prevents the individual from receiving adequate tactile, proprioceptive and kinesthetic stimulation. This reduced stimulation has been postulated as the cause of lower mental functioning.[34]

Given the identified need for sensory stimulation from the environment, and the C.V.A and T.B.I. patient's mobility deficits, which result in limited access to the environment, controlled sensory stimulation is indicated as a primary treatment approach to facilitate patient functioning.

The next concept to consider in applying sensory integrative techniques to adults is brain plasticity. Brain plasticity refers to the adaptive capacities of the central nervous system. It involves the brain's ability to create functional and structural changes when necessary to increase function.[36] Some researchers state that plasticity is accomplished by collateral axonal sprouting, which occurs after brain damage and serves to take over the function of the damaged area.[37,38] The patient with brain damage therefore learns to substitute alternative mechanisms for those he has lost.

It is well documented that a child's normal development involving continuing environmental interaction causes functional and structural brain changes, which in turn allow the child to deal more effectively with the environment. This is accomplished because the brain is considered "plastic" or malleable. Sensory integrative therapy, utilizing the concept of plasticity, is based on the premise that directed environmental interaction with the learning disabled child can result in functional neurological changes. Considerable research in the field has supported this premise.

The concept of brain plasticity in mature adults is controversial. Some professionals believe that there is little or no potential for plasticity in the adult brain. Other professionals believe that there is sufficient potential for plasticity in the adult brain to respond to therapeutic intervention. These professionals believe that regardless of the age of the individual, the central nervous system is dynamic and ever-changing.[39] They believe that there is evidence of some type of plasticity, because functional recovery does occur in brain-damaged adults, even when the lesion is massive and the patient is elderly.[40] Several animal research studies indicate brain plasticity and the potential for the external environment to influence neuroanatomical structures, even in adult organisms.[41,42] Animal research studies have also indicated that an enriched or normal environment slows down and sometimes prevents the decrease in neural functions associated with age.[26] If one believes that brain plasticity does exist in adults, controlled sensory stimulation, followed by adaptive environmental interaction, is indicated as a primary treatment approach.

Although described separately, the concepts pertaining to age, environment and plasticity are related. The C.V.A. or T.B.I. patient suffers losses in all sensory systems, in the vestibular and autonomic nervous systems, and in mobility which results in poor sensory processing and integration. The remediation of the deficits previously described involves concepts related to environment, ie, providing an enriched environment through controlled sensory stimulation. A major underlying concept related to the success in providing this enriched environment is the potential for brain plasticity. Through the brain's potential for plasticity, the elderly C.V.A.

individual or T.B.I. patient is able to register and process sensory stimulation from the environment, undergo functional neurological changes related to this stimulation, and subsequently carry out an adaptive response.

Although the theoretical constructs described appear sound, there remains a paucity of documented studies substantiating the use of sensory integration therapy with the adult brain-damaged patient.

Several studies have been conducted with geriatric blind and hemiplegic adults which profess to apply sensory integration theory to their treatment. Upon examination of these studies, however, it appears that the concepts and techniques applied were not a purely sensory integrative approach. There is one study, however, which does appear sound.

Baker-Nobles and Bink provided sensory integration therapy to blind adults.[43] They hypothesized that sensory integration problems were responsible for the learning problems, postural problems, and self-stimulating behaviors present in the blind individual. They utilized bolsters, net swings, scooterboards, vibration, rubbing, rolling, tilt boards, obstacle courses, and the like as modes of treatment. The results of their study indicated that the sensory integrative therapy provided caused improvement in equilibrium reactions, postural security, bilateral integration, and tolerance of movement in the subjects of the study.

Before concluding this section, two subjects need to be addressed. The first area of concern is that of precautions. Providing sensory integration therapy, and more specifically vestibular stimulation, to the brain-damaged adult can cause nausea, fatigue, dizziness, changes in blood pressure, seizures, and abnormal associated reactions.[29] Measurements of blood pressure and other vital signs should be taken before, during, and after (for up to 24 hours) vestibular stimulation has been provided. The planned initiation of a new technique such as spinning should be communicated to all medical and allied health professionals caring for the patient so that potential problems can be monitored around the clock. Finally, it cannot be stressed enough that the beginning therapist should not attempt to incorporate strong vestibular stimulation, such as rotatory stimulation, into the treatment program unless it is done under the direct supervision of an experienced therapist.

The second area of concern is related to the therapist's knowledge of sensory integration therapy and its relationship to other treatment approaches. Sensory integration theory and application incorporate concepts and techniques which are also contained in approaches such as sensorimotor, developmental or neurodevelopmental.[27] The therapist must understand and remember that "...while sensory integration is considered to be an example of a sensorimotor approach, not all sensorimotor approaches to intervention can be called sensory integration."[27] Without a clear understanding of how sensory integration theory relates to other approaches, its application to the brain-damaged adult is impossible.

Neurodevelopmental Approach

Neurodevelopmental treatment (N.D.T.) is a comprehensive management approach to motor recovery as it relates to activities of daily living.[44] Treatment is aimed at giving the patient control over his movements, with every treatment performed in a functional situation.[45] Balance reactions and the use of the arm and hand for support are facilitated.[45]

The N.D.T. approach works specifically to inhibit abnormal reflex mechanisms and facilitate normal movement.[45] Tactile and kinesthetic stimulation through handling and movement are provided to encourage contact between the individual and the environment.[46] The patient is taught to move normally in all functional tasks. The ultimate goal is to teach the patient how to control his own movements automatically without the aid of the therapist.[47] Movements of the upper and lower trunk are considered key to postural control and limb function, and are therefore facilitated.[27] The therapist works toward the development of a variety of postural sets that make movements easy and automatic.[45] This in turn makes possible the redevelopment of a normal body scheme, leading in turn to improvement in higher level discrimination skills.

Proponents of the N.D.T. approach have recently reanalyzed the basic theoretical concepts in conjunction with what is now known related to motor learning. In a survey of 431 therapists, 89.9% believed that the theoretical concepts of N.D.T. should be revised to include current knowledge related to advances in neuroscience, motor learning, motivation, praxis, etc.[44] The same survey revealed that although many therapists are using handling techniques such as proximal points of control and weight bearing and weight shifts, others are now providing a more family-centered approach, and are encouraging active patient involvement with minimal handling techniques. This shift in emphasis allows the patient to initiate and direct his own movements.

Recent research and theoretical literature related to N.D.T. outlines two new ideas or theoretical assumptions. The first area relates to the concept of "forced use." The term forced use is used to describe the technique of directing the patient's attention and effort to the hemiparetic extremity to the exclusion of the uninvolved limb.[48] By using this technique, the patient can "...never assume a passive role in which motoric responsibility is transiently elicited through the application of external stimuli."[48]

Recent research has shown that the application of forced use can change the functional capacity of even chronic neuro patients.[48] It is hypothesized that through the use of this technique, 1) existing axons and synapses which were previously unused are "unmasked" or made available, or 2) motivation and repetition through the use of existing sensory motor neural circuitry overcame a learned non-use.[48]

The second area of expanded conceptual basis of N.D.T. relates to motor learning and movement analysis. Motor learning is viewed as "...a set of internal processes that are associated with practice or experience."[49] This practice or experience leads to long-lasting or permanent changes in motor behavior. The C.V.A. or T.B.I. patient must relearn movement through functional activities. The therapist must structure activities to enable the patient to relearn and retain the desired goal. Limited feedback is given during the practice of a motor task in order to facilitate maximum retention.[49]

Factors that affect motor learning are movement organization, environmental factors and cognitive processing. If variability of practice of different tasks is experienced by the patient, a stronger, more generalized motor program will be developed.[49] Therefore, practice of functional activities such as transfers or dressing should be practiced in a variety of ways. This will facilitate retention and transfer.

Environmental factors will influence motor learning. Which environmental factors are important will depend on the goal of the action or task. Environmental factors can include areas such as timing or spatial components.

Cognitive processing will also affect motor learning. Patient performance "…in a difficult learning context forces the client to use multiple and variable processes to overcome the difficulty of practice."[49] Performance will be more difficult at the beginning stage when the patient is first acquiring a skill; however, this is beneficial to both retention and learning. Jarus summarizes the key areas to successful motor relearning as follows:

> Contextual variety, open environment, and low knowledge of results … facilitate cognitive motor functioning during motor skill acquisition, thereby enhancing retention and transfer.[49]

The final area of consideration in motor relearning is movement analysis. It is now believed by many therapists utilizing N.D.T. that movement analysis should include all systems which affect movement. These systems include musculoskeletal, synergistic organization, muscle tone, sensation, automatic reflexes, equilibrium and perception/cognition.[50] The components of the movement analysis include the base of support, alignment, sequencing and stability/mobility.[50] The ultimate goal for the patient is efficient functional movement with a large variety of movement options.[50]

In summary, N.D.T. practice still includes many of the original concepts and techniques outlined by Berta Bobath. The theory base however, has recently expanded to include the concept of "forced use" as well as concepts drawn from motor learning such as organization of movement, environmental influence on movement and cognitive processing as it relates to movement performance and analysis.

The use of the neurodevelopmental treatment approach is recommended not only as an effective means of restoring normal motor function, but also as a means of restoring a normal body scheme that ultimately assists in restoring higher level visual perceptual skills. Examples of the uses of neurodevelopmental treatment are described in the sections related to body scheme disorders.

The Affolter Approach

The Affolter approach focuses on "…facilitating perceptual-cognitive representation through problem-solving experience, which is assumed to be at the root of a variety of skills."[51] Affolter believes the tactile-kinesthetic system is crucial to this problem-solving experience.[52,53] In order to learn, the patient must experience learning situations and interact with the environment. The therapist must present to the patient problem-solving tasks such as those he experiences in everyday life.[54]

The Affolter method focuses on input and is process oriented. It is a hands-on functional approach that is based on the belief that the individual will learn best by "doing."[51] The tactile kinesthetic system provides information to the patient related to actions and objects. This in turn leads to perceptual inferences.[53] These perceptual inferences are necessary to effective problem-solving. Effective problem-solving in turn leads to learning and independence.

The goal of treatment utilizing the Affolter approach is based on the premise that the patient must be challenged enough so that learning takes place, but assisted so the patient does not get frustrated.[53] Mistakes are allowed during treatment so that the patient is able to help solve the problem.[51]

The goal is for the patient to reach his optimum level of performance, which is termed "performance ceiling."[51] Davis describes indications that the patient is functioning at his performance ceiling as follows:

1.   Silence while the patient is working
2.   Intent facial expression
3.   Appropriate eye contact
4.   Normal muscle tone

Problem-solving experiences range from simple to complex, and the patient must receive tactile-kinesthetic information during the process.[52,53] The therapist assists the patient in gaining this information through nonverbal guiding. When the therapist provides this guiding, he is facilitating patient exploration and is less concerned with the final outcome of the task. By physically guiding the patient's hands and body in functional activities, the patient can process stimulation without extra stimuli.

Tactile-kinesthetic interaction occurs between the therapist and the patient during guiding.[52] The therapist receives information from the patient, such as changes in tenseness or tone, as he guides. There are three levels of guiding: maximal assist (heavy) and moderate and minimal assist (light).[53] The amount of tactile-kinesthetic information provided depends on body tone, which will change depending on the input or activity.[53] During guiding, the therapist places his hands over the patient's down to the fingertips and guides the correct manipulation of an object.[51] Only the patient's hand should come into contact with the object, and when the therapist feels the patient is taking over the movement, the assistance is reduced.[51] Every time there is a breakdown in movement or hesitation, the therapist resumes guiding as needed.[51,53]

When guiding, the therapist must be sensitive to the patient's movements, and be familiar with the activity in order to anticipate what the patient will experience.[51] Whenever possible, the therapist guides both hands and tries to involve the whole body to challenge posture as well as the upper extremities.[51] The patient's movements should be regular (not too slow, not too fast) and the therapist should provide changes in resistance during the activity.[51,53]

Guiding is initially done in contact with a support reference.[53] For example, the patient's hand is guided along the sink to the faucet during homemaking or grooming activities. When the patient progresses and exhibits normal tone, then guiding can be done without a support base.[53] These movements are more representative of normal movement in daily life.

In summary, the Affolter approach is a process-oriented approach which assumes the individual must interact with the environment in order to learn. The primary means to this learning is tactile-kinesthetic based problem-solving, and environmental exploration, which is facilitated by nonverbal guiding provided by the therapist. Table 1-2 summarizes the key concepts of the frames of reference utilizing the remedial approach.

Table 1-2. Remedial Treatment Approaches (Key Theoretical Concepts)

Approach	Underlying Assumptions
Sensory Integration	Sensory Integration (S.I.) is the organization of sensation for use. S.I. converts our initial sensations into meaningful perceptions. S.I. occurs during an adaptive response.
Neurodevelopmental	Inhibit abnormal reflex mechanisms and facilitate normal movement. Tactile and kinesthetic stimulation through handling and movement is provided to encourage contact between the individual and the environment. The redevelopment of normal postural movement makes possible the redevelopment of normal body scheme, leading to improved perceptual and visual discrimination skills. The use of the "forced use" technique can change the functional capacity of the patient. The patient must relearn movement through functional activities. Factors which affect motor learning are movement organization, environmental factors, and cognitive processing. Movement analysis should include all systems which affect movement.
Affolter	The tactile-kinesthetic system is key to problem solving. Effective problem solving leads to learning and independence. In order to learn, the patient must experience learning situations and interact with the environment. Treatment is process-oriented and focuses on the input.

Frames of Reference Utilizing an Adaptive Conceptual Base

Top-Down Approaches
Occupational Performance (Person-Environment-Performance)

The goal of therapy based on an occupational performance frame of reference is to remediate or reduce dysfunction relating to daily life tasks.[1] Occupational therapy is geared to help the patient develop a sense of competency and self-esteem.[8] Theoretical occupational performance concepts are derived from general systems theory, which views the individual as a whole consisting of many interdependent and related parts. The individual is seen as a living open system which can exist only if there is ongoing interaction between the individual or environment. This interaction should subsequently create change in both the systems as well as the environment. The relationship of the open system and the environment is viewed as a performance transaction.[55] This performance, when described in the context of daily living skills, is termed occupational performance. Occupational performance is the "...doing part of real life occupation in self-care, play, leisure, and work."[5] The three levels of occupational performance are activities, tasks and roles. Activities consist of outlined steps and are analyzed in relation to requisite abilities.[1] An individual's ability is the result of genetic make-up and learning. These abilities are used to master new skills or "task proficiency."

Tasks consist of four dimensions that have differing degrees of structure, complexity and purpose, and are temporal in nature. Tasks are sets of activities which the individual believes share the same purpose, and are larger units of behavior than activities.[1,8] An individual's role varies depending on the time in his life. Competence is achieved by meeting the responsibilities of a given role in order to perform daily living tasks. A state of "occupational dysfunction" occurs when there is a breakdown in the ability to perform life's roles.

Occupational performance can be affected depending on the individual, the environment and/or the task itself. Environments which can alter performance include social, cultural, and "arousal environment." An individual's arousal environment or level of awareness will influence his inclination and ability to explore his surroundings. There are three occupational performance components related to occupational function. These components are sensorimotor, cognitive and psychosocial.[8] Subserving these components are various subskills or enablers. For example the subskills of the performance component of cognition would include arousal, orientation, recognition, attention span, memory, sequencing, categorizing, concept formation, problem solving, and the "...generalization, integration and synthesis of new learning."[5] Each of these subskills can be broken down further. For example, memory is composed of areas such as sensory memory, procedural memory or episodic memory.

Trombley summarizes well the goals of an occupational performance approach. Occupational function occurs when the patient:[8]

1. Gains a sense of efficiency and therefore feels competent.
2. This competence is derived from being in control of one's life and therefore having the ability to satisfactorily engage in a chosen life role.
3. To satisfactorily engage in a life role, one must be able to do the tasks that make up that role.
4. Tasks are made up of activities which are smaller units of behavior.
5. To be able to do an activity one has to have certain sensorimotor, cognitive, perceptual, emotional and social abilities.
6. Abilities are developed from capacities that the person has gained through practice or maturation, or both.
7. These developed capacities are the person's genetic make-up or spared organized systems.

Functional Approach

The functional approach is a top-down approach which works directly with actual occupations.[5,8,12,56] It uses functional or occupation tasks to maximize the patient's independence. The functional approach emphasizes the patient's strengths and can be domain specific (repetitive practice of a specific functional task) and/or involve specific adaptations or compensation.[12] The desired outcome of the functional approach is effective adaptation.[5] Effective adaptation always occurs within an environmental context, therefore, a variety of functional activities are practiced in different environments. The functional approach utilizes two major categories of techniques: compensation and adaptation.

Compensation

In the compensation approach, the patient is made aware of his problem and then taught to compensate, or make allowance for it. For example, if the patient neglects one-half of space because of unilateral neglect, one would teach him to turn his head or scan with his eyes to the affected side. Or if he had dressing apraxia, one would practice a particular dressing pattern with him daily.

Adaptation

Adaptation usually goes along with compensation. In this approach, one makes changes in or adapts the environment of the patient to compensate for his symptoms. For example, if he tends to neglect one-half of space, the therapist would put all of his food and utensils on the unaffected side to be sure that it is seen. If the patient has figure-ground problems, the therapist would try to unclutter the environment to make it easier to locate objects. If the patient has topographical disorientation, the therapist would mark the route to be followed every day. Informing the patient's family about his problems so that they can make allowances for them, instead of thinking that the patient is stubborn or crazy, is a more subtle form of adaptation. Adapting the patient's "human" rather than his "nonhuman" environment is of major importance in many ways.

The functional approach is one of the most favored in the clinic today. Recent research has supported its use for improved self-care of patients with unilateral neglect or perceptual dysfunction.[56] Rubio and Van Deusen, however, found that for wheelchair mobility and driving, a combination of functional and restorative was the most effective approach.[56] An additional benefit of the functional approach is its relevance to the patient. Patients often object to abstract perceptual and cognitive training, finding it childish, degrading, and not relevant to their problems.

One final benefit of utilizing a functional approach relates to the status or focus of today's health care. The trend for shorter hospital stays and the need for specific expedient measured outcomes, necessitates the use of an approach which can meet these demands. Often a restorative approach to treatment requires extended stays, which has become less and less an option.

Dynamic Interactional Approach*

Central to the Dynamic Interactional Theory (D.I.T.) is the concept that cognition is an ongoing production or outcome of the interaction between the individual, the task and the environment.[57] The patient's performance is analyzed by examining the underlying conditions and processing strategies that change performance. Evaluation and treatment are carried out in a variety of situations, or contexts (multi-context). The goal of multi-context learning is to improve the patient's ability to "...process, monitor and use new information flexibly across task situations."[57]

D.I.T. examines the patient's ability for change.[59] Assessment includes task alteration and cues strategy training, practice in a number of settings, and the examination of learner characteristics to facilitate learning transfer.[57] Assessment is focused on the patient's ability to: 1) evaluate the level of difficulty of a particular task, 2) plan ahead, 3) select appropriate strategies, 4) predict the consequences of the actions he takes and 5) monitor performance.[57]

The above skills are defined as "metacognition" and are paramount to the generalization of new learning. Metacognitive skills are related to both motivation and past experience. If a patient believes he has some degree of control of his performance, his motivation will increase. This emotional state of mind will in turn influence how well information is processed and monitored.[58] Past experience guides how the patient processes and organizes information.[57] When new information is processed by relating it to previous knowledge, understanding and retention improve.

In addition to environmental considerations, D.I.T. focuses on task analysis. Toglia[59] divides tasks into both surface and conceptual characteristics. Surface characteristics are those characteristics which are readily observed. Conceptual characteristics, on the other hand, cannot be directly observed. These characteristics would include areas such as the strategies used to perform the task or what the task means to the patient. Toglia states that "...by analyzing the task's characteristics, one can understand the conditions that cause information processing to break down."[57] This type of task analysis differs from the deficit specific approach in which the inter-relationship between cognitive skills during processing and task performance is not described.

In addition to examining the patient's potential for change, assessment focuses on the patient's best performance and what task and environmental criteria are needed to achieve this performance. If a patient has difficulty, test procedures are changed and subsequent patient response is examined. Treatment application of the D.I.T. and multi-context concepts involves "...practicing targeted processing strategies and self-monitoring techniques in a variety of situations and environments."[57] Tasks are analyzed and upgraded to place additional demands on the impaired processing system and the ability to transfer new learning.[57] A variety of activities including tabletop, computer, functional and gross motor activities are used. Treatment begins at the level of breakdown and the task is not upgraded until there is some evidence that generalization of learning has occurred at the highest level of transfer.[60] Task, strategy and metacognitive training are performed in a variety of settings, with the ultimate goal of learning transfer.

---

*The Dynamic Interactional Approach can be viewed as both a remedial and adaptive approach. Some treatment alters the task or environment more than the person, however, ultimately the D.I.A. is changing the person and how he performs the task (personal communication Joan Toglia, MA, OTR). For the purposes of this book, the approach and related treatment ideas will be described under the adaptive approach.

TABLE 1-3. ADAPTIVE TREATMENT APPROACHES
(KEY THEORETICAL CONCEPTS)

Approach	Underlying Assumptions
Occupational Performance	The individual as an open system exists through the interaction between the individual and the environment. This relationship between the individual and the environment is a performance transaction. The three levels of occupational performance are activities, tasks and roles. Activities require certain sensorimotor, cognitive, perceptual, emotional and social abilities. To satisfactorily engage in a life role and achieve competence, one must be able to do the tasks that make up the role.
Functional	Functional tasks retraining is utilized to maximize patient independence. Patient is made aware of his problem and taught to compensate for it, and/or the environment or task is adapted to maximize function.
Dynamic Interactional	Patient is made aware of his problem and taught to compensate for it, and/or the environment or task is adapted to maximize function. Patient performance is analyzed by examining the underlying conditions and processing strategies that change performance. Evaluation and treatment are carried out in a variety of situations or contexts (multi-context). Multi-context learning promotes generalization and use of information and strategies across task situations.

Table 1-3 summarizes the key concepts of the frames of reference utilizing the adaptive approach.

References

1. Christiansen C. Occupational therapy: Intervention for life performance. In: Christiansen C, Baum C (eds.). *Occupational Therapy: Overcoming Human Performance Deficits.* New Jersey, SLACK Inc.; 1991.

2. Mosey AC. The paper focus of scientific inquiry in occupational therapy: Frames of reference. *Occupational Therapy Journal of Research*. 1995;9(4):195-201.

3. Mathiowetz V. Role of physical performance component evaluations in occupational therapy functional assessment. *Amer Journal of Occup Ther*. 1993;47(3):225-230.

4. Titus MLD, Gall NG, Yerxa EJ, Roberson TA, Mack W. Correlation of perceptual performance and activities of daily living in stroke patients. *Amer J Occup Ther*. 1991;45(5):410-417.

5. Abreu B, Duval M, Gerber D, Wood W. Occupational performance and the functional approach. AOTA Self Study Series: *Cognitive Rehabilitation*. The American Occupational Therapy Association, Inc.; 1994.

6. Abreu B, Toglia J. Cognitive rehabilitation: A model for occupational therapy. *Amer J Occup Ther*. 1987;41(7):439-448.

7. Butler RW, Namerow NS. Cognitive retraining in brain-injury rehabilitation: A critical review. *J Neuro Rehab*. 1988;2:97-101.

8. Trombly C. Anticipating the future: Assessment of occupational function. *Amer J Occup Ther*. 1993;47(3):253-257.

9. Ben-Yishay Y, Diller L. Cognitive Deficits. In: Griffith E, Bond M, Miller J (eds.). *Rehabilitation of the Head Injured Adult*. Philadelphia, FA Davis; 1983.

10. Farrel W, Schultz-Krohn W. A computer program for enhancing visuomotor skills. *Amer J Occup Ther*. 1990;44(6):557-559.

11. Fordyce DJ. Neuropsychologic assessment and cognitive rehabilitation: Issues of psychologic validity. In: Finlayson MAJ, Garner SH (eds.). *Brain Injury Rehabilitation: Clinical Considerations*. Baltimore, Williams and Wilkins; 1994.

12. Neistadt ME. A critical analysis of occupational therapy approach for perceptual deficits in adults with brain injury. *Amer J Occup Ther*. 1990;44:299-304.

13. Sohlberg MM, Mateer CA. *Introduction to Cognitive Rehabilitation: Theory and Practice*. New York, The Guilford Press; 1989.

14. Wood RL. A neurobehavioral approach to brain injury rehabilitation. In: VonSteinbuchel N, VonCramon DY and Poppel E (eds.). *Neuropsychological Rehabilitation*. Berlin, Springer-Verlag; 1992.

15. Neistadt ME. Assessing learning capabilities during cognitive and perceptual evaluations for adults with traumatic brain injury. *Occup Ther in Health Care*. 1995;9(1):3-16.

16. Tankle RS. Application of neuropsychological test results to interdisciplinary cognitive rehabilitation with head-injured adults. *J Head Trauma Rehabil*. 1988.3(1):24-32.

17. Zemke R. Task skills, problem solving, and social interaction. In: Royeen CB (ed.). AOTA Self Study Series: *Cognitive Rehabilitation*. American Occupational Therapy Association, Inc.; 1994.

18. Dougherty PM, Radomski MV. *A Dynamic Assessment Approach for Adults with Brain Injury: The Cognitive Rehabilitation Workbook*. Gaithersburg, MD, Aspen Publishers; 1993.

19. Neistadt ME. A meal preparation treatment protocol for adults with brain injury. *Amer J Occup Ther*. 1994;48(5):431-438.

20. Radomski MV, Dougherty PM, Fine SB, Baum C. Case studies in cognitive rehabilitation. In: Royeen CB (ed.). AOTA Self Study Series: *Cognitive Rehabilitation*. American Occupational Therapy Association, Inc.; 1994.

21. Allen CK. Treatment plans in cognitive rehabilitation. *Occup Ther Pract*. 1989;1(1):1-8.

22. Bruce MAG. Cognitive rehabilitation: Intelligence, insight, and knowledge. In: Royeen CB (ed.). AOTA Self Study Series: *Cognitive Rehabilitation*. American Occupational Therapy Association, Inc.; 1994.

23. Ayres AJ. *Sensory Integration and Learning Disorders*. Los Angeles, Western Psychological Services; 1980.

24. Cabay M, King LJ. Sensory integration and perception: The foundation for concept formation. *Occup Ther Pract*. 1989;1(1):18-27.

25. Jongbloed LE, Collins JB, Jones W. A sensorimotor integration test battery for CVA clients: Preliminary evidence of reliability and validity. *Occup Ther J Res*. 1986;6(3):131-150.

26. Ayres AJ. *Sensory Integration and the Child*. Los Angeles, Western Psychological Services; 1980.

27. Fisher A, Murray EA, Bundy AC. *Sensory Integration: Theory and Practice*. Philadelphia, FA

Davis; 1991.

28. Arnadottir G. *The Brain and Behavior: Assessing Cortical Dysfunction Through Activities of Daily Living.* St. Louis, CV Mosby; 1990.

29. Zoltan B, Ryckman D. Head injury in adults. In: Pedretti (ed.). *Occupational Therapy for Physical Dysfunction.* 2nd ed. St. Louis, CV Mosby; 1985.

30. Moskowitz E, Lightbody EEH, Freitag NS. Long term follow-up of the post stroke patient. *Arch Phys Med Rehab.* 1972;53:167-172.

31. Crovitz H. Memory retraining in brain-damaged patients: The airplane list. *Cortex.* 1979;15:131-134.

32. Kenshalo DR. Changes in the vestibular and sonmesthetic systems as a function of age. In: Ordy JM, Bizzee KR (eds.). *Aging. Vol. 10. Sensory Systems and Communication in the Elderly.* New York, Raven Press; 1979.

33. Ordy JM, Brizzee KR. Sensory coding: Sensation perception, information processing, and sensory-motor integration from maturity to old age. In: Ordy JM, Bizzee KR (eds.). *Aging. Vol 10. Sensory Systems and Communication in the Elderly.* New York, Raven Press; 1979.

34. Sawtell R, Martin G. Perceptual problems of the hemiplegic patient. *Lancet.* 1967;87:193-196.

35. Solomon P, et al. *Sensory Deprivation.* Cambridge, Harvard University Press; 1961.

36. Restak R. *The Brain.* Toronto, Bantam Books; 1984.

37. Bach-y-Rita P. *Recovery of Function: Theoretical Considerations for Brain Injury Rehabilitation.* Bern, Hans Huber Publishers; 1980.

38. Geschwind N. Late changes in the central nervous system: An overview. In: Stein D, Rosen J, Bulters N (eds.). *Plasticity and Recovery of Function in the Central Nervous System.* New York, Academic Press, Inc.; 1974.

39. Drachman D, Leavitt J. Memory impairment in the aged: Storage vs. retrieval deficit. *J Exp Psychol.* 1972;93(2):302-308.

40. Layton B. Perceptual noise and aging. *Psychol Bull.* 1975;82:875-883.

41. Diamond MC. The aging brain: Some enlightening and optimistic results. *Am Scient.* 1978;66:66-71.

42. Rosensweig MR. Environmental complexity, cerebral change and behavior. *Am Psychol.* 1966;21:321-332.

43. Baker-Nobles L, Bink MP. Sensory integration in the rehabilitation of blind adults. *Am J Occup Ther.* 1979;33(9):559-564.

44. DeGangi GA, Royeen CB. Current practice among neurodevelopmental treatment association members. *Amer J Occup Ther.* Sept 1994;48(9):803-809.

45. Bobath B. *Adult Hemiplegia: Evaluation and Treatment.* London, William Hennemann Medical Books Ltd.; 1978.

46. Davies PM. *Steps to Follow—A Guide to the Treatment of Adult Hemiplegia.* Berlin, Springer-Verlag; 1985.

47. Meltzer M. Poor memory: A case report. *J Clin Psychol.* 1983;39(1):3-10.

48. Wolf SL, Lecraw DE, Barton LA, Jann BB. Forced use of hemiplegic upper extremities to reverse the effect of learned nonuse among chronic stroke and head-injured patients. *Exper Neurology.* 1989;104:125-132.

49. Jarus T. Motor learning and occupational therapy: The organization of practice. *Amer J Occup Ther.* Sept 1994;48(9):810-816.

50. Fisher B, Yakura J. Movement analysis: A different perspective. *Orthopedic Physical Therapy Clinics of North America: The rehabilitation setting.* Mar 1993;2(1):1-14.

51. Davis ES, Radomski MV. Domain-specific training to reinstate habit sequences. *Occup Ther Pract.* 1989;1(1):79-88.

52. Affolter FD. *Perception, Interaction and Language; Interaction of Daily Living: The Root of Development.* Berlin, Springer-Verlag Co.; 1987.

53. Bonfils K. Affolter Approach. In: Pedretti L (ed.). *Practice Skills for Physical Dysfunction.* St. Louis, CV Mosby; 1995.

54. Affolter F, Stricker E. *Perceptual Processes as Prerequisites for Complex Human Behavior: A Theoretical Model and its Application to Therapy.* Bern, Hans Huber Publishers; 1980.

55. Duchek J. Cognitive dimensions of performance. In: Christiansen C, Baum, C (eds.). *Occupational Therapy: Overcoming Human Performance Deficits.* Thorofare, New Jersey, SLACK Inc.; 1991.
56. Rubio KB, Van Deusen J. Relation of perceptual and body image dysfunction to activities of daily living of persons after stroke. *Amer J Occup Ther.* 1995;49(6):551-559.
57. Toglia JP. A dynamic interactional approach to cognitive rehabilitation. In: Katz N (ed.). *Cognitive Rehabilitation: Models For Intervention in Occupational Therapy.* Boston, Andover Med Pub.; 1992.
58. Brown AL. Motivation to learn and understand: On taking charge of one's own learning. *Cognition and Instruction.* 1988;5:311-321.
59. Toglia JP. Generalization of treatment: A multicontextual approach to cognitive perceptual impairment in the brain injured adult. *Amer J Occup Ther.* 1991;45(6):505-516.
60. Toglia JP. Approaches to cognitive assessment of the brain-injured adult: Traditional methods and dynamic investigation. *Occup Ther Pract.* 1989;1(1):36-57.

CHAPTER 2

General Evaluation Issues

Before the evaluation of visual, perceptual and cognitive processing abilities can be initiated, several general evaluation issues must be taken into consideration. These issues include test reliability and validity, administration of tests, test scoring, qualitative versus quantitative analysis and evaluation choice.

Test Reliability and Validity

A test's reliability refers to its consistency and accuracy. Reliability can be measured in several ways. One way is to administer a test to an individual several times. If the score is approximately the same over repeated examinations, the test-retest reliability is said to be good. By repeating this procedure with a large group of people, one can perform a statistical analysis and derive a coefficient of correlation r for the test. A test's test-retest correlation r can range from 0 to 1.0. The higher the r, the better the test-retest reliability. If a test has a test-retest correlation of 0.60 or higher, it is considered fairly reliable. One should be sure that a test has a fairly high test-retest correlation if one intends to use the test as a measure of improvement following treatment.

Scorer or inter-rater response is another method of measuring a test's reliability. Here two or more examiners score a set of tests and their results are compared. The closer the sets of scores are to each other, the better the test's scorer reliability. Again, the range of the coefficient of correlation r is from 0 to 1.0, and the closer it is to 1.0, the better. The results of tests of reliability are usually found in a test's manual.

Unless the criteria for making the judgment for score assignment is explicit on a subjective test, the scorer reliability of the test is likely to be low. Therefore, it is difficult to compare results between patients or between testings of the same patient if the tests are scored by different examiners. However, since anyone giving an objective test should get the same results as anyone else, the scorer reliability is likely to be high. It still may not be a reliable or consistent test; it's test-retest reliability may be low.

Only a few of the objective visual, perceptual or cognitive tests have been standardized for adult populations, although some have been standardized for children. A standardized test is defined as any test that has been administered to a large sample of the population one wishes to test so that the examiner knows how the average person in this population scores on this test. When tests have not been standardized, interpretation of scores is tenuous, since there are no norms for comparison.[1,2] In such instances, it is suggested that if one is unfamiliar with the test and with how the normal adult will perform, it should first be administered to several normal adults, preferably of the same age, sex, and occupational or educational level as the patient. In this way, one can develop skill in test administration and gain some idea of how well a normal adult should score on the test.

The validity of many of these tests has not been examined. A test's validity refers to how well the test measures what it purports to measure. There are several types of validity. One type—content validity—describes how well the test represents the total universe of the content of the property being measured.[3] Deciding the degree to which it does this is basically a matter of judgment. However, other types of validity can be measured by statistical analysis. The results of such tests are usually found in a test's manual. Although many of the tests reported here have content validity, their total validity has only occasionally been statistically established. For this reason, a low score on any one test is not conclusive evidence that the patient has that particular deficit. A low score on one test should signal the need for follow-up with a series of similar tests.

Only a few studies have been done to correlate results of tests of perception and cognition with actual functional abilities and disabilities. This is part of examining the test's validity. For example, an adult patient may do very poorly on *Ayres' Figure-Ground Test,* yet have no observable functional deficit in that area. Those perceptual or cognitive tests that have been shown to correlate with functional performance will be specified when each specific deficit is described. The problem of lack of research to correlate test scores and functional performance has led some occupational therapists to rely solely on functional tests, eg, can a patient dress himself, rather than on formal perceptual or cognitive tests. The problem that functional tests present is that one cannot always discern why the patient is having trouble doing the task. One can hypothesize reasons and then test them with the more discrete formal visual, perceptual and/or cognitive tests. In this way, a combination of functional and perceptual or cognitive tasks can be most useful.

Administration of Tests

In administering the tests described in the following chapters, one should be aware of several additional problems. First, none of these tests measure completely discrete functions. They may emphasize one main function, but most overlap into other areas. To use these tests with greater validity, one must first rule out other deficits the patient may have. For example, in testing tactile agnosia, the inability to recognize objects by touch although sensation is intact, one must first test to be sure that the patient has normal tactile sensation. Throughout the test descriptions, under the heading "To Improve Validity," those deficits that may interfere with performance on a particular test should be tested first. Unfortunately, other deficits may be an inherent part of the test and thus be impossible to completely rule out. For example, a right hemiplegic patient and a left hemiplegic patient may perform equally poorly on a constructional praxis test, but for entirely different reasons. The right hemiplegic tends to have trouble initiating or carrying through the construction, which is more an execution problem; the left hemiplegic tends to pick up and move blocks around randomly, which is more a spatial relations problem.[4] Therefore, the examiner must be aware of the different causes of poor performance on a given test and look closely at the qualitative performance by the patient for clues to the reason for his failure.

Second, all the tests require comprehension of the directions, and some require verbal responses. Thus their use with aphasic patients must take this into account. These tests may not be valid for aphasics; they may measure language rather than perceptual or cognitive skills.

Third, many of the tests require some motor act as part of the response. Patients should first be tested for apraxia and lack of motor control to rule out problems in the areas in the tests at which a motor response is required.

Fourth, although the patient appears to be mentally alert, he may do poorly on these tests because he is inattentive or easily distracted. This may be the result of brain damage. According to Luria,[5] lesions in the frontal lobe affect a patient's ability to form intentions or goals, to attend and concentrate. The patient may be inattentive because the task is too abstract for him. Hague[6] showed that left hemiplegics have a definite impairment of complex abstract behavior and should be tested on the concrete level. Or a patient may have a very short immediate visual memory, making it difficult for him to attend to the task.

Vision is also a factor in many of these tests. Often patients who have sustained a C.V.A. are elderly and have poor eyesight that is not always corrected well by their glasses. This should be checked before administering tests in which visual acuity is important. Information about aging, vision, and visual evaluation and treatment are covered in detail in Chapters 3 and 11.

A patient's pre C.V.A. or T.B.I. intelligence, perceptual and cognitive skills, and educational and cultural background can also affect his performance. For example, if a patient was developmentally delayed before a C.V.A. or T.B.I., he will have difficulty with some abstract concepts in the tests even if there are no perceptual or cognitive problems as a result of the insult or trauma. Or if the patient's background is such that he never learned to write or draw, paper and pencil tests may not be valid. Or if, for various reasons, he never developed his perceptual or cognitive skills to their fullest capacity, low scores on the tests would not necessarily be the result of a C.V.A. or T.B.I.

Lastly, one may get poor results because the patient reacts negatively to this type of testing. He may find the tasks childish and refuse to do them. The patient may think that they are intelligence tests and become very anxious about performance. For this reason the therapist must be careful in explaining the purpose of all tests.

Test Scoring

If the test has been standardized, it is important to administer it exactly according to the accompanying directions in order to use the test's norms. Any standardized objective test can, however, also give subjective or qualitative information depending on how data are collected. For example, the standardized procedures may be utilized but the patient's approach to the task and patient verbalizations may also be recorded.[7]

Three categories of tests are examined in this manual. They are:

1. Standardized—scored objectively, standardized with adults.
2. Nonstandardized—scored objectively, not standardized with adults.
3. Subjective—scored subjectively, not standardized.

In scoring subjective and nonstandardized tests, a patient's performance is usually labeled intact, impaired, severely impaired, or absent. An intact performance is defined as the way a normal adult would perform on the test. A severely impaired/absent performance is defined as one in which the patient is making many errors, taking longer than normal to do the test, or having trouble completing the test. An impaired performance is between a severely impaired and an intact performance. The patient completes the test but makes one or two errors, or does not perform the task quite correctly.

In the following chapters, an intact performance will be described on those tests scored subjectively or nonstandardized. If the patient's performance is not intact, the labeling of his performance as "impaired" or "severely impaired" will at times be left up to the examiner, since the difference between the two is one of degree of impairment.

When some tests are used to evaluate more than one deficit, a description of an impaired performance will be included to distinguish qualitative differences of performance between patients with different deficits. For example, a *Copy Flower, House Test*, in which the patient is asked to copy a drawing of a house and a flower, is used to test for both unilateral neglect and constructional apraxia. In order to differentiate between the two deficits when the test is examined during evaluations for unilateral neglect, a description of how a patient with unilateral neglect would perform is included.

Qualitative Analysis Versus Quantitative Scoring

When administering any test or evaluating any task performance, it is important to remember that there is usually more than one reason for failure. It is often just as important to understand *why* the patient has failed as the actual score.[8] Qualitative analysis of the patient's performance goes beyond specific performance data and should be collected along with quantitative information.[9]

Specific quantitative measures include accuracy measures (number of errors, percentage correct, number correct), time (speed of performance, rate of responding), and cuing (amount of cuing, type of cuing used, number of self corrects, etc.).[10] Qualitative measures include internal factors such as depression, level of confidence or distraction. It also includes measures of external factors such as noise or interruptions. Distinctive error patterns such as errors grouped at the beginning, throughout or the end of therapy are also measured. Sohlberg and Mateer provide the following information pertaining to common error patterns:[9]

*   Increased errors over time: inadequate sustained attention, fatigue factor
*   Increased errors at the beginning of a task: difficulty picking up a new task or poor mental flexibility
*   Many errors throughout the task: inability to understand the directions or simply can't do the task.

Evaluation Choice

There are many factors to consider in deciding which evaluation to utilize. This manual contains descriptions of multiple evaluation tools for each area described and **it is not intended for the therapist to administer all evaluations**! Factors such as aphasia, motor and visual ability, patient setting, and occupational performance status will all play into the ultimate decision. Outside pressures such as reimbursement, cost of materials and therapist time will also have to be considered. Finally, patient response, the theoretical support for the technique, and the therapist's ability to administer the test adequately should also be considered.[11]

References

1. Boys M, Fisher P, Holzberg C, Reid DW. The OSOT perceptual evaluation: A research perspective. *Amer J Occup Ther.* Feb 1988;42(2):92-98.
2. VanDeusen-Fox J, Harlowe D. Construct validation of occupational therapy measures used in CVA evaluation: A beginning. *Amer J Occup Ther.* Feb 1984;38(2):101-106.
3. VanDeusen-Fox J, Harlowe D. Continued construct validation of the St. Mary's CVA evaluation: Bilateral awareness scale. *Amer J Occup Ther.* April 1987;41(4):242-245.
4. Harrington DO. *The Visual Fields.* 4th ed. St. Louis, CV Mosby; 1976.
5. Luria AR. Functional organization of the brain. *Sci Am.* 1970;222:66-72.
6. Hague HR. An investigation of abstract behavior in patients with cerebral vascular accidents. *Am J Occup Ther.* 1959;13:83-87.
7. Milberg WP, Herben N, Kaplan E. The Boston process approach to neuropsychological assessment. In: Grant I, Adams KM (eds.). *Neuropsychological Assessment of Neuropsychiatric Disorders.* New York, Oxford University Press; 1986.
8. Ratcliff G. Perception and Complex Visual Process. In: Meir MJ, Benton AL, Diller L. *Neuropsychological Rehabilitation.* New York, Guilford University Press; 1987.
9. Sohlberg M, Mateer CA. Effectiveness of an attention-training program. *J Clinical Exper Neuropsych.* 1987;9(2):117-130.
10. Sohlberg MM, Mateer CA. *Introduction To Cognitive Rehabilitation: Theory and Practice.* New York, The Guilford Press; 1989.
11. Okkema K. *Cognition and Perception in the Stroke Patient.* Gaithersburg, Aspen Publishers; 1993.

CHAPTER 3

Visual Processing Skills

Vision plays a major role in our ability to adapt to the environment. A large portion of our daily life requires effective visual processing and visuo-motor performance.[1] It is an important prerequisite to perception and cognition and influences both motor planning and postural control. It allows us to anticipate information, which is necessary for successful adaptation to the environment.[2] Visual deficits can have a great impact on ADL, reading, driving and eye-hand coordination.[3] Without an efficient level of visual function, the rehabilitation process is adversely affected.[4]

Visual processing occurs through two modes: focal control or attentive vision, and ambient, peripheral or pre-attentive vision.[2,5-7] Focal vision provides attention to important features of an object for perception and discrimination. Ambient vision works in connection with proprioceptive, kinesthetic, tactual and vestibular systems and acts as a feed-forward system.[6] In order for the focal visual process to function effectively, the ambient process must initially organize and stabilize the visual field. Peripheral or ambient vision detects events in the environment and their location in space and distance from the individual.[2] It monitors verticality of objects and body alignment with them. Ambient vision is also the mode of vision which ties into functional mobility.[8]

Visual deficits sustained subsequent to C.V.A. or T.B.I. may be due to a "dysfunction of the ambient process in its ability to organize spatial information with other sensory-motor systems."[6] This inability in turn will cause a compromise to the focal process. Successful adaptation requires that both the ambient and focal systems work together, and that the visual system as a whole be integrated with other sensory input.

Some clinicians view visual processing through a general information processing theory.[1] The first, or *input*, stage of processing is affected by the integrity of the optical system or eye health, a clear optical image, the intact functioning of the accommodative and convergence systems, good fusional ability and efficient oculomotor control. During the second, or *integrative*, stage of processing, sensory and proprioceptive information are mixed. This blending or combination of information results in a concept or plan that will serve as a guide to an action or response.[1] The final, or *output*, stage of processing involves the integration of the "ocular motor response, the accommodative convergence relationship, fusional and accommodative facility and visuo-motor integration."[1]

An alternative view to visual processing which has recently gained popularity with therapists involves the concepts of a hierarchy of visual processing and a view of visual processing as a process of adaptation.[2] Visual information processing is viewed as an interactive product of both bottom-up and top-down processing.[5] Vision and visual processing are viewed holistically as a "single, unified process used by the central nervous system to adapt."[2] Visual processing occurs within a hierarchy of skills rather than a series of independent skills. At the most basic level is registration of visual input through oculomotor control, visual fields and acuity. This is followed by visual attention, organized scanning, pattern recognition and visual cognition.[2] Visual cognition is an end product of all preceding skills and is the highest level of visual skill integration within the nervous system. Any inefficiency in the lower level skills such as scanning, or visual fields, will alter the patient's ability to "...cognitively apply these skills to adapt."[2]

The evaluation and treatment of the patient's visual ability should incorporate both the component skills and how the system as a whole is working. The therapist should examine where in the visual hierarchy the breakdown of performance is occurring, evaluate what conditions cause a breakdown in the adaptation process, and determine what changes can be made within the task and environment to improve performance.[2] In addition, "...we must also develop our own style of intervention and determine the unique contribution that occupational therapists can make to this field."[9]

Evaluation of Visual Skills

Due to the impact of visual processing deficits on all other areas of function, the evaluation and treatment of these deficits should be handled early in the rehabilitation process.[7]

General Guidelines for Visual Processing Skills Evaluation

Clinical Observations[2]

Observe for possible indications of visual stress such as shutting an eye, squinting, increased muscle tone in head and jaw, turning or cocking the head, changing head position during ambulation, complaints of headaches or fatigue, or sudden agitation when a task is presented.

1. Do the eyes work together?
2. How well do the eyes work together?
3. Where is the visual control most and least efficient?
4. What kinds of eye movements are the most and least efficient?
5. How does altering the environment or task alter performance?

Specific Component Skills to Evaluate

It is not the occupational therapist's role to perform an extensive eye examination. It is, however, his responsibility to obtain from the optometrist or ophthalmologist necessary information related to areas such as glaucoma, or other medical conditions related to eye health. The same factors that cause brain damage can also cause damage to the eye itself.[10]

The clinical evaluation of certain component skills within the hierarchy of visual processing and how they affect functional adaptation is well within the occupational therapist's role. Included in the evaluation are ocular alignment, oculomotor control (saccadic eye movements, smooth pursuit movements), convergence, visual attention/scanning, visual memory and visual cognition. In addition, if a vision specialist, optometrist or ophthalmologist is immediately unavailable, an acuity screening is indicated.

Visual Acuity

Visual acuity is the end product of the integration of the optical systems of the eye and central nervous system processing.[2] Impaired acuity can be the direct result of a C.V.A. or T.B.I.[11] Without intact or corrected visual acuity, effective spatial resolution is not possible.

The three most common optical defects are myopia (nearsightedness), hyperopia (farsightedness), and astigmatism. In addition, the patient may have difficulty with visual processing in environments with low contrast sensitivity.[2] Normal visual acuity is 20/20, with a minimum of 20/40 required for driving.[11] Distance acuity deficits will affect the patient functionally in areas such as depth perception, spatial judgments and facial recognition.[11,12] Near vision deficits will affect reading, writing and any other functional activities requiring "close work."[11,12]

Evaluation of Visual Acuity

The optometrist, ophthalmologist or vision specialist should do a complete acuity evaluation. If these disciplines are not immediately available, the occupational therapist should conduct an acuity screening. This evaluation should be done prior to all other visual testing.

General Guidelines for Evaluation

1. Distance acuity is tested initially at 20 feet. Near acuity is tested at 4 cm or 16 inches.[13]
2. The patient should wear glasses during the evaluation if he or she normally does so.
3. A tumbling E chart, Landolt C chart or the Lighthouse Picture symbols test are especially useful with the aphasic patient.[4]
4. For the patient with severe visual perceptual problems, modify the testing by presenting one visual stimulus at a time and direct the patient's eye to the stimulus by pointing.[5]

Visual Acuity Screening

TEST 1: DISTANCE VISUAL ACUITY[3*]

Purpose:
To test clearness of vision at distance.

Vision problems detected:
Loss of vision, reduced vision due to uncorrected refractive condition (myopia, hyperopia, astigmatism), amblyopia (lazy eye), etc.

---

*Reproduced with permission from Lynn Hellerstein, OD, Homestead Park Vision Clinic, P.C., 6967 S. Holly Circle, Suite 105, Englewood, CO, 80112.

Control:
Habitual glasses for distance, if worn by patient. Patient may be seated or standing at the appropriate distance from the chart (varies with each other). Make sure lighting is adequate.

Equipment:
Distance acuity chart (Snellen, pictures, tumbling E, Broken Wheel) occluded.

Procedure:
Test the right eye first, occlude left eye. Ask the patient to read the smallest letters (or picture). If the patient reads the line correctly, proceed to the next smaller line. Don't allow the patient to squint. Encourage "guessing." If the patient has difficulty, isolate letters. Continue until the patient misses letters. Once completed, switch occluder to right eye and test left eye, then both eyes. Always watch the patient, not the chart.

Recording:
Write down the ratio listed next to the smallest line read. If patient missed any letters on that line, record the ratio minus the number of letters missed (eg, if patient read four of six letters on the 20/20 line, record as 20/20-2). If the patient must move to ten feet to read off a chart meant to be used at 20 feet, record as test distance/smallest line read (eg, if patient could see the 20/100 letters at ten feet, record as 10/100).

Retest/referral:
Patient should be able to read at least 20/30 with each eye. 20/40 acuity or worse is a referral.

TEST 2: NEAR VISUAL ACUITY[3]*

Purpose:
To test clearness of vision at near (within arm's length).

Vision problems detected:
Vision loss, reduced vision due to uncorrected refractive error, accommodation dysfunction, etc.

Control:
Habitual glasses for near, if worn. Make sure lighting is adequate.

Equipment:
Near visual acuity card (letters, picture, etc.).

Procedure:
Hold card at appropriate distance (as noted by each card, usually 13 or 16 inches). Test right eye first. Procedure is same as for distance visual acuity.

Re-test/referral:
Patient should be able to read 20/20 or better with each eye. 20/40 or worse is referral.

TEST 3: PEPPER VISUAL SKILLS FOR READING TEST[14]

Description:
The Pepper Visual Skills for Reading Test (VSRT) provides an accurate and reliable estimate of the patient's ability in the visual components of the reading process. It is primarily designed for use with patients with macular disease, which creates central scotomas, which inhibits reading ability. The VSRT measures the following component skills:

1.   Visual word recognition ability
2.   Saccadic and return sweep eye movement control

---

*Reproduced with permission from Lynn Hellerstein, OD, Homestead Park Vision Clinic, P.C., 6967 S. Holly Circle, Suite 105, Englewood, CO, 80112.

3. How well the patient can position the central scotoma so that it doesn't obscure the field of view necessary for reading

The test is arranged in order of difficulty, timed and individually administered in approximately 10-15 minutes. It contains fifteen rigid cards printed in size five print. The cards have unrelated letters and words on them.

Scoring:
The VSRT provides both accuracy (mean percentage correct for each completed line) and rate (correct words per minute) measures. The type of errors made are also recorded.

Reliability:
Pearson-product moment correlation for accuracy measures was .90 (p<.01). Pearson-product moment correlation for rate scores was .97 (p<.01).

Validity:
Correlation measures between the VSRT and Gray Oral Reading Test were taken. Pearson-product moment correlation for the reading rates of both tests was .82 (p≤.05).

Treatment of Visual Acuity

If screening indicates impairment, initiate a referral to an ophthalmologist or optometrist for continued evaluation, prescription lens or additional treatment as needed.

Utilizing an Adaptive Approach:

1. If acuity cannot be corrected with lenses, utilize enlarged print, control the density of presented stimuli, utilize contrast and lighting.[15]

2. If the patient appears to have difficulty processing visually under conditions of low contrast or illumination, provide environmental adaptation as follows:[2,16,17]

   a. Increase contrast—for example, bright tape on stairs, bright paint on doors, cabinets, bright labels on prescriptions, canned goods, etc. Use light walls with dark furniture, light switch plugs and electrical outlets. Vertical blinds and shades can help control the amount of light in a room.

   b. Increase light with minimum glare through halogen or fluorescent lighting. Reduce shadows by avoiding single bulb or recessed lighting. Filters or absorptive lenses can be incorporated into prescription lenses. Non-glare paper or a sheet of yellow acetate can be placed over a page of print. Visors and side shields can also be used if glare is a problem. For near tasks, the light should be placed on the side of the best eye or opposite the working hand.

   c. Utilize solid colors for rugs, bedspreads, dishes, countertops, etc. Patterns can blend with the background and cause decreased object identification.

   d. Decrease clutter in the environment, i.e. cabinets, closets, countertops, etc. Self-threading needles and magnetic padlocks which do not require a combination can also help.

   e. For writing, bold tip pens or markers can be used to make large letters. Bold line paper, stand magnifiers, closed circuit televisions that provide magnification of the writing area, typewriters, and computers can all be used as needed.

f.   Motion lights which turn on automatically when someone enters a room or dark hall-way can help prevent falls.

g.   To compensate for visual loss, utilize the remaining sensory systems (hearing, tactile discrimination, kinesthesia proprioception) to assist in increased function.[9] Also, have the patient rely on language to interpret form and space.[18]

3.   Provide treatment in a variety of "contextually" relevant environments.

4.   Applying an occupational performance frame of reference, identify the areas of occupational performance which are affected by the changes in visual performance.[9] Warren outlines five key areas which are addressed in the treatment plan:[9]

a.   Efficient and effective use of optical devices to read materials needed for daily living

b.   Ability to write legibly to complete communications needed for daily living

c.   Ability to complete financial transactions and manage financial affairs independently

d.   Ability to complete self-care and homemaking activities with optimum efficiency, independence and safety

e.   Ability to engage in leisure and community activities

Ocular Alignment

Ocular alignment is crucial to the coordinated function of both eyes and visual processing in general. If both eyes are not aligned, the patient may experience double vision (diplopia), vertigo, confusion, clumsiness, motion sickness, and/or poor spatial judgment.[15]

Evaluation of Ocular Alignment

TEST 1: HIRSCHBERG TECHNIQUE[19]

Procedure:
Patient fixates on a penlight held directly in front of him. Observe the reflection of the light on the corneas of both eyes.

Scoring:
If the eyes are evenly aligned, the reflection will appear in the same location in each pupil.
Esotropia:
One eye is deviated inward; the reflection will occur on the lateral aspect of the pupil in that eye.

Exotropia:
The reflection will be observed on the medial side of the pupil.

Treatment of Deficits in Eye Alignment

There are numerous underlying causes of decreased eye alignment. If the screening indicated a problem, a referral should be made to an optometrist, ophthalmologist, or vision specialist.

Utilizing a Remedial Approach:

1.   If it is established by the optometrist, ophthalmologist or vision specialist that the problem

is due to a muscle imbalance, then eye exercises can be initiated. Active range of motion exercises should be done in the direction of the paresis (Warren, personal communication).

2. If the patient is experiencing double vision, provide: a) occlusion and b) activities to obtain fusion. For example: provide a control target at the distance the patient can obtain fusion. Gradually move the target away to have the patient maintain fusion at a further distance (Warren, personal communication).

Visual Fixation

The ability to visually attend is present in elementary form at birth and matures by four weeks. For the normal adult, visual fixation is a voluntary act. The normal adult has no difficulty in selecting objects within his environment and focusing his gaze upon them.

The adult C.V.A. or T.B.I. patient may have difficulty in visually attending to objects within the environment. The deficit may be an inability to obtain fixation or the inability to sustain it. It may be associated with or occur separately from spatial or body neglect or inattention.

Evaluation for Visual Fixation

TEST 1: WARREN[2]

Procedure:
Evaluate the patient's ability to locate and fixate on a target in various locations within the visual fields as follows. Present target first at midline and then to the right and left of midline at near (16-20") and middle (21-36") focal distances.

Scoring:
Patient should be able to locate the target, fixate on it and maintain fixation for several seconds.

Treatment for Visual Fixation

Treatment for visual fixation is generally addressed with scanning due to their close connection (Warren, personal communication). Tasks can include letter recognition through reading, progressing to more difficult tasks such as paragraph reading.

Visual Fields

The normal monocular field of vision is approximately 60 degrees upward, 60 degrees inward, 70 to 75 degrees downward, and 100 to 110 degrees outward. The type of deficit the patient sustains depends on location and size of the lesion. Deficits may include homonymous hemianopias, quadrantopias, scotomas (areas of decreased sensitivity) and/or visual constrictions.[15] Visual field deficits may be seen in patients with or without associated visual neglect. Patients do generally exhibit small saccadic eye movements, decreased speed of scanning (particularly with saccades toward the impaired field) and a narrower scope of scanning.[2,20]

Functional deficits associated with visual field loss are numerous and diverse. A few examples include reading, finding objects, dressing, and visual memory.[2,11,20] Warren[2] identifies the

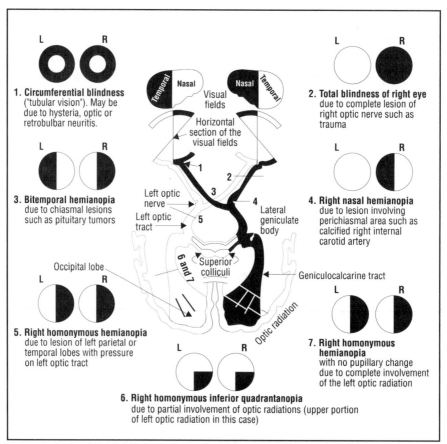

1. **Circumferential blindness** ("tubular vision"). May be due to hysteria, optic or retrobulbar neuritis.

2. **Total blindness of right eye** due to complete lesion of right optic nerve such as trauma

3. **Bitemporal hemianopia** due to chiasmal lesions such as pituitary tumors

4. **Right nasal hemianopia** due to lesion involving perichiasmal area such as calcified right internal carotid artery

5. **Right homonymous hemianopia** due to lesion of left parietal or temporal lobes with pressure on left optic tract

6. **Right homonymous inferior quadrantanopia** due to partial involvement of optic radiations (upper portion of left optic radiation in this case)

7. **Right homonymous hemianopia** with no pupillary change due to complete involvement of the left optic radiation

Labels within figure: Visual fields; Temporal; Nasal; Horizontal section of the visual fields; Left optic nerve; Left optic tract; Lateral geniculate body; Superior colliculi; Occipital lobe; Geniculocalcarine tract; Optic radiation

Figure 3-1. Visual field deficits and associated lesion sites. Reproduced with permission.

following four factors which will influence whether field loss will affect overall function:

1. Whether the field cut is homonymous or congruous in each eye.
2. The contour of the boundary between the sound and scoptic field (ie, if the boundary is abrupt, the patient has more difficulty compensating).
3. The presence of a control field cut.
4. Patient's awareness of the field cut.

The types of common visual field deficits and associated lesion sites are illustrated in Figure 3-1.

Evaluation of Visual Field Cuts

The most accurate measure of visual fields is computerized automated perimetry. If this is unavailable then confrontation testing is recommended.[4,21-24] The results of confrontation testing should be interpreted in combination with the patient's performance with activities of daily living.

TEST 1: CONFRONTATION TESTING WITHOUT EYE PATCH*[25]

Both eyes together: The therapist sits directly in front of the patient, about 18 inches away. The patient fixates on the examiner's nose. If possible, the patient's back should be to the light with the patient facing a dark uniform background behind the examiner. The test objects are two dull black 2-foot wands with white balls on the end. When testing with both wands together, the therapist is checking for the extinction phenomenon. The therapist alternates using one or two wands and moves either or both in from the right or left periphery, at times simultaneously, in the simulated arc of the visual fields, meeting in the center, toward fixation. The patient is asked to indicate whether he sees one target or two while he focuses on the examiner's nose. He is also asked where they are located. The therapist should alternate the pattern by presenting one target in the right field, one in the left, and then both together. Repeat for a total of nine times. The target should be moved again in the three planes: eye level, forehead and below chin level (three times each level).

Directions:
1. (*Verbal Patient*) "I want you to keep both eyes on my nose. Tell me if you can see one ball or two and where it is located. You can point to where it is if you wish. Do you see one ball or two? Where?"
2. (*Nonverbal Patient*) "Before I tell you what to do, I want you to keep both eyes on my nose. Tell me if you see one ball or two by pointing to the one(s) you see. Do you see one ball or two? Point to what you see."

Scale:
1- Present, visual field loss noted.
0- Absent, no visual field loss noted.

TEST 2: CONFRONTATION TESTING WITH EYE PATCH*[25]

Each eye separately: The therapist sits directly in front of the patient, about 18 inches away. The patient fixates on the examiner's nose with one eye while the other eye is covered with an eye patch. If possible, the patient's back should again be to the light, and there should be a dark uniform background behind the examiner. The test object used is a white ball on the end of a dull black 2-foot wand.

The test object is moved in from the periphery of the patient's field (from the left and then the right) in an arc simulating the curve of an imaginary sphere (perimeter).

The object is moved slowly in at eye level first, and then repeated at forehead level and just below chin level (nine times). The patient is asked to respond verbally or with a gesture as soon as he can see the target. The eye patch is then switched and the test repeated on the other eye.

Directions:
1. (*Verbal Patient*) "For this test I want you to keep your eye on my nose. Say yes as soon as you see this white ball move in from the side."
2. (*Nonverbal Patient*) "For this test, I want you to keep your eye on my nose. Raise a finger (or hand) as soon as you see the white ball move in from the side."
3. Observe whether there is sufficient visual attentiveness for this test and the quadrants of each eye in which the patient has difficulty in attending to stimuli. The problem can be central, peripheral, or anywhere in the field.

Scale:
1- Present, visual field deficit noted.
0- Absent, all visual fields intact.

Reliability:
Both the described confrontation tests, when given alone (ie, not in conjunction with addi-

---

*Reproduced with permission from Santa Clara Valley Medical Center, San Jose, CA.

tional visual skills testing), did not reach an acceptable level (ie, r>0.75) of inter-rater reliability in a study conducted on a sample of patients who had sustained head trauma. However, these tests, utilized as part of an overall visual skills evaluation, did have good inter-rater reliability (r=0.82 for overall visual skills evaluation). In addition, inter-item correlations between the two tests revealed an almost perfect correlation (r=0.97). This almost perfect correlation suggests that administering both tests (ie, with and without the patch) provides no additional information. Further research should indicate whether deleting one of these tests is justified in order to shorten the evaluation.

Confrontation testing, similar to the tests described, is commonly utilized as a measure of visual fields in the adult patient with head trauma. To improve validity, rule out aphasia, poor visual attention, and scanning as causes of poor performance.

Treatment of Visual Field Deficits

Utilizing a Remedial Approach:

1. Place a bedside table, comb, newspaper and any commonly used objects on the side of poor vision, forcing the patient to look to that side.
2. Provide verbal, auditory (bell, finger snapping) and tactile cuing to encourage the patient to look to the affected side.
3. Practice worksheets as described in the treatment of visual scanning and unilateral neglect.
4. Provide the patient with computer retraining, utilizing software specifically designed for the remediation of visual field deficits.
5. Some researchers believe that visual retraining involving light sensitivity measures and measures of saccadic localization in deficit fields can actually increase visual function.[20] These findings, however, were not replicated in similar studies.[26]

Utilizing an Adaptive Approach:

1. Place all necessary items for functional independence within the patient's field of vision.
2. Educate the patient and his family about his field loss and how it will potentially affect function. Situations where safety may be a problem should be highlighted.
3. If possible, have the patient identify his own compensation strategies and provide a variety of tasks which allow the patient to apply these strategies. Carry out the tasks in a variety of contexts or environments.

Oculomotor Control

Oculomotor control is crucial to the efficient processing of visual information. Oculomotor deficits are common after brain damage and can vary depending on the size and location of the lesion. Decreased oculomotor control results in slower speed, control and coordination of eye movements with a subsequent disruption of visual scanning and attention.[2] Deficits can severely impair the patient's ability to effectively scan his environment, and in turn devastate him functionally. Oculomotor control consists of saccadic eye movements or fixations and smooth pursuit movements.

Saccadic Eye Movements

Saccadic eye movements are sequenced rapid eye movements that change the line of sight. These movements place an object of interest on the fovea of the eye.[2] Saccadic eye movements involve the use of peripheral vision. By consciously "turning off" one's peripheral vision, saccadic eye movements become more efficient and organized. Saccadic eye movements are used extensively in reading.

Evaluation of Saccadic Eye Movement

TEST 1: KING-DEVICK TEST[27]

Description:
This test consists of one demonstration card and three test cards. (Figures 3-2 through 3-4). Subtest I consists of randomly spaced numbers connected by horizontal lines; Subtests II and III do not include any lines.
The patient is asked to call out numbers in order as fast as possible, following the arrows.

Scoring:
The time for completion is recorded in whole seconds, and the number of errors is noted for each subtest.
This test has established norms (sample=1202) for ages 6 to 14.
To improve validity, rule out impaired visual attention and aphasia as causes of poor performance.

TEST 2: WARREN[2]

Procedure:
Hold two objects several inches apart and ask the patient to first fixate on one target and then the other. Hold the targets approximately 16" from the bridge of the nose.

Scoring:
The patient should be able to smoothly shift his gaze between the two objects without turning his head.

TEST 3: BOUSKA[15]

Procedure:
The patient looks rapidly from one object to another. The two objects are held approximately 6 inches apart about 12-15 inches from the patient.

Scoring:
A slight overshoot, undershoot or refixation of the target may be within normal limits. Large errors should be considered abnormal.

TEST 4: PEPPER (VRST)[14]
Refer to this test in the section for the evaluation of visual acuity.

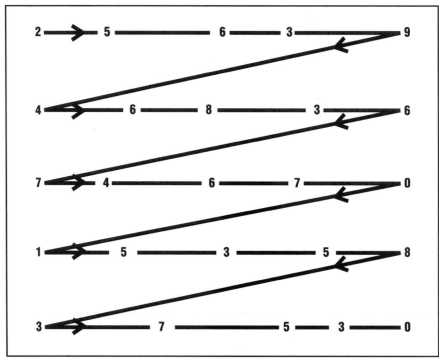

Figure 3-2. King-Devick Demonstration Card. Reproduced with permission from the Bernell Corp., PO Box 4637, South Bend, IN.

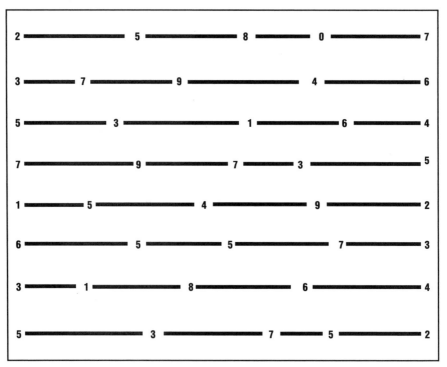

Figure 3-3. King-Devick Test I. Reproduced with permission from the Bernell Corp., PO Box 4637, South Bend, IN.

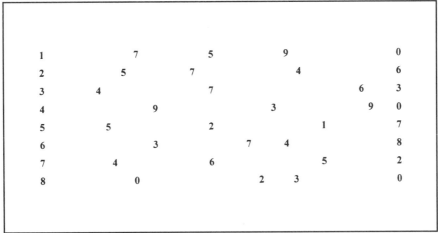

Figure 3-4. King-Devick Test II. Reproduced with permission from the Bernell Corp., PO Box 4637, South Bend, IN.

Treatment of Deficits in Saccadic Eye Movements

Utilizing a Remedial Approach:

1. Have the patient perform such activities as calling out or pointing to letters from two columns printed on either side of a page (Figure 3-5). To progress with the activity, the column of printed letters should be printed closer to the center of the page (Figure 3-6). This activity can be adapted further by placing the columns on a blackboard and changing the distance between the columns as the patient progresses.
2. Provide vestibular based movement activities in conjunction with demands for saccadic skills. For instance, have the patient roll one-quarter turn and identify a number or letter that has been randomly placed on a suspended ball. Repeat the activity with a half turn, a three-quarter turn, and so on.
3. Provide computer retraining utilizing software designed specifically for the remediation of basic oculomotor deficits.

Utilizing an Adaptive Approach:

1. Provide anchoring during reading tasks.
2. Control the density of the visual information being presented.

Smooth Pursuit Eye Movements

Smooth pursuit eye movements are those movements that keep an image steady on the retina. These movements track a moving object when the head is stationary. An impairment in smooth pursuit eye movement often results in a pursuit movement supplemented by saccades.[15] This jerky interruption of smooth pursuits is considered abnormal.

1F		T1
2N		U2
3P		P3
4V		X4
5R		A5
6M		W6
7H		F7
8O		B8
9S		Z9
10T		L10
11K		E11

Figure 3-5. Saccadic Eye Movement Worksheet 1.

1X		C1
2M		T2
3A		W3
4F		B4
5O		L5
6Z		H6
7P		N7
8W		S8
9C		X9
10G		R10
11N		V11

Figure 3-6. Saccadic Eye Movement Worksheet 2.

TEST 1: DIRECTION OF GAZE

Description:

All six muscles that move each eye (the four rectus muscles—superior and inferior, lateral and medial—and the two oblique muscles—superior and inferior) are tested. The therapist asks the patient to "look first to one side and then to the other" to test the medial and lateral rectus muscles. While looking to the one side, the subject is instructed to look up and down; in this position, the adducted eye is elevated by the superior rectus muscle and depressed by the inferior muscle. The abducted eye is elevated by the inferior oblique muscle." Repeat the procedure with the opposite side to test the opposite muscles.

Scoring:
Nonstandardized.
Intact: The patient is able to direct his gaze in all directions as requested.
Impaired: The patient is unable to direct his gaze in one or more directions requested.
(Specify which movements are impaired.)
Unable to perform: The patient is unable to direct his gaze in any direction as requested.
To improve validity, rule out aphasia and poor performance.

TEST 2: OCULAR PURSUITS*[12]

Description:
The therapist moves an orange rubber ball on the end of a dowel back and forth approximately 18 inches in front of the patient's eyes at eye level. The object is moved two or three times slowly in each direction in this order: horizontally, vertically, diagonally (right to left and left to right), clockwise and counterclockwise.

Directions:
"Follow this ball with your eyes in the direction I move it. Move only your eyes and not your head."
Observe for short visual attention span, abnormal jerky eye movements, and excessive head movement. Observe whether the patient loses track of the object or cannot follow in a smooth pursuit. Note nystagmus, particularly at the end of eye movement range or at midline. Again note convergence of eye gaze, difficulty in crossing midline, overshooting, and whether a full range of motion of eye movement is present.

Scoring:
2- Absent, unable to track a moving object.
1- Impaired, has difficulty tracking a moving object in any or all directions.
0- Intact, eyes smoothly follow in all directions.
To improve validity, rule out aphasia and poor visual attentiveness as causes of poor performance.

Reliability:
This test has established inter-rater reliability (r=1.0) with a sample of adult patients sustaining head trauma.

Organized Scanning

TEST 1: SCANBOARD TEST
Developed by Mary Warren MS, OTR in collaboration with members of the Occupational Therapy Department, Eye Foundation of Kansas City, 2300 Holmes Street, Kansas City, MO 64108.

Purpose:
The patient is able to employ an organized and symmetrical strategy in scanning for visual information. Research with the test has shown that normal adults will employ an organized sequential scanning pattern to identify the numbers on the board using one of three patterns: clockwise, counterclockwise or rectilinear. Most individuals will start in the upper left hand corner and scan left to right and top to bottom.*
For further information regarding the test see: Warren ML. Identification of visual scanning deficits in adults after cerebrovascular accident. *Amer J Occup Ther.* 1990;44:391-399.

---

*Reproduced with permission from Santa Clara Valley Medical Center, San Jose, CA.

Test Materials:
- Scanboard
- Easel

Instructions:
1. The patient should be seated in a posturally secure position with good midline orientation (straddling the low bench is best). The board should be at eye level in the patient's midline and within arm's reach so the patient can touch each number on the board.
2. Instructions to the patient: "There are 10 numbers on this board. Point the numbers out to me as you see them. Do not go in any particular order—just point them out as you see them. Point slowly because I will be writing down the numbers you see. Begin."
3. On the score sheet, indicate on the line under each number the order in which it was identified.
4. Do not cue the patient during the test—let him indicate to you when he is finished.
5. On completion, analyze the scanning pattern for organization (see examples).

Treatment for Organized Scanning

Utilizing a Remedial Approach:

1. Develop strategies with the patient on how to take in visual information in an organized manner. Train the patient to attend to spatial details.
2. Have the patient perform an activity for which effective scanning is required to complete the activity, but is not the focus of the activity.[28]
3. Have the patient perform tasks such as the following:
   a. Cross out target letters (eg, all A's) in the paragraph of a magazine, newspaper article, or scanning worksheet designed by the therapist. Utilize the retraining principles of anchoring, pacing, density, and feedback (see Number 1 below).
   b. Complete paper mazes, puzzles, or other activities that require scanning ability.
4. Have the patient perform functional tasks which require scanning, such as:
   a. Have the patient scan his room or clinic for specified items.
   b. Take the patient to a community setting, such as a grocery, department, drug, or hardware store. In a particular section of the store, have the patient locate and retrieve a set of items listed by the therapist.
   c. Locate names, items, and prices, as specified by the therapist, in the classified ads of the newspaper.
   d. Locate names, numbers or addresses in a local telephone directory.

Utilizing an Adaptive Approach:

1. Provide the patient with the following adaptations and cuing:[28-30]
   a. Anchoring or cuing the patient as to where to begin the visual search. For example, red tape or marker can be placed to the left at the beginning of all lines to be read or scanned.
   b. Pacing or cuing the patient about the speed of his response. This will help control impulsive or erratic scanning and establish an appropriate scanning rate. Slowing the

patient down can be accomplished simply by having him call out each number or letter as it appears, or by placing a sticker under each one that is called out.[30]

   c. Controlling the density or spacing of visual stimuli.[30] In other words, change the distance between adjacent stimuli.

   d. Providing consistent feedback to the patient about his performance of visual scanning tasks. The patient is progressed by gradually decreasing any of the cues.

2. For activities such as dressing, utilize an audiotape with instructions and stack clothes in a consistent order.[31]

3. Educate the patient and his family about the scanning deficit and how it will affect function. Highlight areas where safety will be an issue.

Convergence

Normal convergence is essential for effective near vision. Cohen et al[32] define convergence as "the simultaneous and synchronous adduction movement of the eyes resulting in an increased angle between the visual axes." Convergence requires the integration of both cortical and subcortical functions. In a study of 26 brain-injured patients, convergence insufficiency was correlated with overall rehabilitative outcome as evaluated by actual work placement.[32]

Decreased accommodation or convergence will lead to symptoms and stress for the patient.[4] The patient may complain of fatigue with reading, writing, crafts, or any other activities requiring close focal distance.[2]

Evaluation of Convergence

TEST 1: WARREN[2]

Procedure:
The patient follows a target with his eyes in toward the bridge of his nose.

Scoring:
Normal.
The patient is able to maintain binocular fixation on a target to approximately 3 inches of the nose.

TEST 2: PADULA ET AL[6]

Procedure:
A .5 cm silver steel ball supported by a black rod is moved in toward the patient's nose. Convergence ability is recorded at the point of reported diplopia or loss of ocular alignment. Recovery is the point at which the patient reports single vision or when ocular alignment is noted.

Scoring:
Absent—no convergence.
Impaired—inability to converge on the target within 12 cm working distance.
Intact—convergence less than 12 cm working distance.

TEST 3: NEAR POINT OF CONVERGENCE (NPC)[3]*

Purpose:
To screen for adequate convergence (aiming) skills.

Vision problems detected:
Convergence insufficiency

Control:
Habitual glasses, if worn by the patient. Be sure patient is looking through near prescription (you might need to lift glasses higher to utilize bifocal and prevent the patient from tipping his head back).

Procedure:
Start with the fixation target at 20 inches from the patient's face. Instruct the patient to stare at the target as you move it slowly toward the patient's nose and to report if the target breaks into two (doubles). As you move the target toward the patient's nose, watch both eyes. If one eye stops converging, the patient might report seeing two targets, and you will see one eye wander outward. Where the tester sees the patient's eyes no longer converge together is called the break point (may be different than where the patient reports double vision). Now slowly bring the target back out. Instruct the patient to report when the target jumps back into one, and observe when the eyes regain fixation. This is called the recovery point. Repeat the test several times to note whether the patient fatigues over time.

Recording:
Write the break point/recovery point (ex: 4/6 inch). If the patient can converge to the nose, record TN (to nose).

Re-test/Referral:
Patient should be able to converge within 6 inches from the bridge of his nose, and recover within 6 inches of the bridge of his nose. Outside this range is a referral.

Visual Spatial Inattention

Visual spatial inattention can be defined as a condition in which there is a decreased awareness of the body and spatial environment on the side contralateral to the cerebral lesion, despite the absence of a specific sensory deficit.[15,33,34] Visual spatial inattention is most common and more severe following right hemisphere lesion,[35-37] can occur with or without the presence of visual field deficits, and may be seen in conjunction with body neglect. Body-centered neglect is associated with frontal lesions, while environment-centered neglect is associated with parietal lesions.[32]

The patient may ignore one of two objects held in intact visual fields on either side of the midline when presented simultaneously. Visual neglect may occur not only for midline opposite stimuli, but for contralateral upper and lower quadrants as well. For example, a lower left quadrant stimulus can cause a simultaneous stimulus in the upper right quadrant to be neglected.

Some clinicians have noted a lack of systematic exploration within the extra personal space. Bouska et al observe that eye movement, both scanning and saccades during activities occurs on only one side of midline within the attended space. This phenomenon occurs in the absence of apraxia for eye movements and with no decrease in extra ocular movements.[15]

---

*Reproduced with permission from Lynn Hellerstein, OD, Homestead Park Vision Clinic, P.C., 6967 S. Holly Circle, Suite 105, Englewood, CO, 80112.

The theoretical basis of visual spatial inattention remains somewhat controversial. Some believe it is due to the interaction between a sensory deficit and mental deterioration.[11,23,35] Others attribute the deficit to an impairment of the internal representation of space.[38] Many believe visual spatial inattention is at least in part due to disordered attention and/or orienting systems.[11,34,35,39,40] Butter[34] builds on the concept of an attention related deficit and divides attention into two categories: reflex and voluntary. Reflex attention is triggered by stimuli with certain physical characteristics. The speed and frequency with which the stimulus has occurred also determine the degree to which it captures our attention of stimuli."[34]

Voluntary attention, on the other hand, "involves the central activation of stored representations of stimuli."[34] It is assumed that voluntary attention is related to neural structures that are located at higher cortical levels and are superimposed on the mechanisms of reflex attention.[34,41] Theoretically, reflex attention involves bottom-up processing of visual stimuli, whereas voluntary attention utilizes both top-down and bottom-up processing.

Riddock and Humphrey[40] support the concept of two types of attention, which they term pre-attentive and attentive processing. Their research indicated that pre-attentive processing appeared relatively intact in a portion of their patients, and therefore they believe that neglect results from an inability to "translate the information pre-attentively into a form which will support action."[40] It is a breakdown in the processes whereby visual stimuli "capture visual attention."

Functional implications for the patient with visual spatial inattention are varied and often severe. Patients will have difficulty with reading, writing, drawing and basically any or all areas of ADL, depending on the severity of deficit.[21,42]

Evaluation of Visual Spatial Inattention

TEST 1: BEHAVIORAL INATTENTION TEST (BIT)[43]

Description:
The BIT is an objective behavioral test of everyday skills relevant to visual neglect. It has nine behavioral subtests and six conventional pencil and paper subtests. Conventional subtests include line crossing, letter cancellation, star cancellation, figure and shape copying, line bisection and representational drawing. The behavioral subtests are picture scanning, telephone dialing, menu reading, article reading, telling and setting the time, coin sorting, address and sentence copying, map navigation and card sorting.

Scoring:
In each subtest the number of omissions is recorded. In addition, errors of commission and/or other types of errors are noted but not incorporated into the score. The total score from the conventional subtests determines the presence of unilateral visual neglect. Behavioral subtests can then be used to identify how the neglect is causing everyday problems and as a guide in treatment strategy. Detailed information on scoring is contained in the test manual.

Reliability:
1. Inter-rater reliability was established at .99 (P<0.001)
2. Parallel form reliability was established between two test versions at .91 (P<0.001)
3. Test-retest reliability was established at .99 (P<0.001).

Validity:

1. A comparison of scores on the behavioral battery to those on the conventional tests was made. The correlation was .92 (P<0.001).
2. Behavioral scores were compared with a short questionnaire completed by the therapist at the time of assessment. The correlation was .67 (P<0.001).
3. Forty Israeli subjects (C.V.A.) were evaluated with BIT, performance tasks and a check-list of ADL. Results supported the construct and predictive validity of most of the BIT subtests as functional measures of unilateral neglect.[44]

Procedure:

The instructions for two of the conventional subtests and two of the behavioral subtests are presented as examples.

Conventional Subtests

LINE CROSSING[43]*

Description:

Subjects are presented with a page containing 40 one-inch (25mm) lines. The page is placed directly in front of them. The lines appear to be randomly spaced about the page but are in fact grouped into three columns containing six lines on either side of the midline.

Instructions:

"On this page we have many lines pointing in different directions. Follow my pen as I indicate these lines." (Move pen right to left, top to bottom over all the lines on the page.) "Now with this pen, I want you to cross out all the lines which you can see on the page, like this." (Illustrate by crossing out two of the four central lines.)

Some patients may initially cross out only those lines which appear to correspond to the orientation of the example. In such cases the patient should be instructed to cross out all the lines, irrespective of orientation.

Scoring:

The total number of lines crossed is noted. The maximum is 36 (18 left, 18 right). The four lines of the central column are not scored.

STAR CANCELLATION[43]*

Description:

Subjects are presented with a page containing 52 large stars, 13 randomly positioned letters and 10 short words, interspersed with 56 smaller stars.

Instructions:

"This page contains stars of different sizes. Look at the page carefully—this is a small star. Every time you see a small star, cross it out like this." (Illustrate by crossing out the two small stars immediately above the centralizing arrow on the stimulus sheet.) "I would like you to go through this page and cross out all the small stars without missing any of them."

---

*Reproduced with permission from Thames Valley Test Co., 7-9 The Green, Flempton, Burry St. Edmunds, Suffolk, England, 1P286E1: Distributed by Northern Speech Services, 117 Elm Street, P.O. Box 1247, Gaylord, Michigan, 49735.

Scoring:
The total number of small stars canceled is noted. The response sheet can be further divided into six sections by the scoring template for further analysis of omissions. Total number of stars is 54 (27 left, 27 right).

Behavioral Subtests

ARTICLE READING[43]*

Description:
The subject is presented with a short, three column article and is instructed to read it. (This is obviously not appropriate for some language impaired patients).

Instructions:
"Here is a short article from a newspaper. Please read it out loud, slowly and carefully."

Scoring:
This is based on the percentage of words omitted in all three columns. Word omission, incomplete words, partial or whole substitutions of words are scored. The examiner uses a photocopy of the original article to record the relevant errors made.

COIN SORTING[43]*

Description:
The subject is presented with an array of coins (six denominations in all, three of each denomination). He is asked to indicate the coins according to the denomination called out. This is arranged according to a pre-set order.

Instructions:
"Here we have a selection of coins which I would like you to look at. There are three rows altogether" (indicate). "I am now going to call out various names of coins and I'd like you to point to the coin or coins I name. Be sure to point out all the coins of each type called out."

Scoring:
All coins identified are recorded on a score sheet. The score is based on the number of omissions. Location of omissions can be noted on the score sheet.

TEST 2: ALTERNATING SIMULTANEOUS STIMULI[25]†

Procedure:
The therapist is seated at arm's length directly facing the patient. The patient is instructed to focus on the therapist's nose. Using the index fingers of both hands approximately eight inches in front of the patient's face, the therapist wiggles one or two fingers two times, a total of seven to 10 trials.

X= Finger moves
0= Finger does not move

Ask the patient to indicate which finger he sees moving, by either pointing or a verbal response.

---

*Reproduced with permission from Thames Valley Test Co., 7-9 The Green, Flempton, Burry St. Edmunds, Suffolk, England, 1P286E1: Distributed by Northern Speech Services, 117 Elm Street, P.O. Box 1247, Gaylord, Michigan, 49735.

†Reproduced with permission from Santa Clara Valley Medical Center, San Jose, CA.

Note: The rating should not overlap with the patient's field cut, as you would be sketching field loss and not neglect. Test for neglect within the patient's visual and on the border of the field deficit if present.

Directions:
"For this test, keep your eyes on my nose at all times. Tell me how many fingers I move—one or two. Point to what moved."
Observe whether the patient is able to attend consistently to visual stimuli presented simultaneously or whether he neglects right or left stimuli.
Note: Visual confrontation on only the affected side may reveal no apparent neglect. However, subsequent simultaneous confrontation may show visual neglect of stimuli in the presence of intact peripheral vision.

Scale:
1- Present, visual spatial neglect noted.
0- Absent, attends to visual stimuli correctly.

TEST 3: LINE BISECTION TEST[45]*

Procedure:
Using the two line bisection worksheets placed and taped end to end directly in front of the patient with the taped section at midline on the table, ask the patient to draw a short line through the middle of each one of the lines (use a pen). Choose a line in the middle of the page to demonstrate. Do not give clues regarding whether the patient has marked all of them, and do not allow movement of the paper. Save the sheet, and mark where the top of the page is.

Time:
90 seconds for the whole task (use as a guideline).

Directions:
"Draw a short line through the middle of each one of the lines that you see. Watch me; this is what I want you to do. Begin." (Do not give clues.)
Observe whether the patient's lines are constantly off midline or whether he draws all the lines on one side of the paper first, and whether he completely misses one area of the page. Poor performance may indicate hemianopsia, visual neglect, poor visual scanning, or all these problems.

Scale:
2- Severely impaired: any mark over 1/2 inch off midline, any missed line, greater than 90 seconds.
1- Minimally impaired: any mark over 1/4 inch off midline, greater than 90 seconds.
0- Intact: all marks within 1/4 inch of the midline, within 90 seconds.
To improve validity, rule out aphasia, decreased visual attention, and scanning and visual field deficit as causes of poor performance.

Reliability:
Tests similar to the ones described have traditionally been used as tests of visual neglect.
The line bisection test, when given as an isolated test, did not reach an acceptable level ($r<0.75$) of inter-rater reliability in a study conducted on a sample of head trauma patients. However, this test utilized as part of an overall primary visual skills evaluation, did have good inter-rater reliability ($r=0.82$ for overall primary visual skills evaluation).

---

*Reproduced with permission from Santa Clara Valley Medical Center, San Jose, CA.

Treatment for Visual Inattention

Utilizing a Remedial Approach:

1. Fresnel Prisms have been shown to reduce visual inattention on visual perceptual tasks.[46] Note, however, that more research is indicated to see if this improvement generalizes to activities of daily living.
2. Some researchers indicate a reduction of visual inattention utilizing monocular patching combined with lateralized stimulation in a line bisection task.[47]
3. Some researchers indicate the use of dynamic stimuli (eg, flashing lights), versus static stimuli, to be effective in the reduction of visual inattention.[34,48]
4. Research has indicated that visual inattention is a result, at least in part, of decreased orientation and attention. Therefore, activities which activate spared brainstem components of this system can significantly reduce inattention.[34]
5. Provide verbal, auditory (bell, finger snapping) and tactile cuing to encourage the patient to look to the unattended space.
6. Provide computer retraining with software designed specifically for the remediation of visual inattention.

Utilizing an Adaptive Approach:

1. Increase the patient's and family's awareness of the visual inattention and how it will affect the patient functionally. Activities where safety is an issue should be highlighted. Also emphasize the need for visual scanning during activities.
2. If possible, have the patient identify his own compensation strategies and provide tasks which allow the patient to apply these strategies. Carry out the tasks in a variety of contexts or environments.
3. Emphasize visual scanning activities and show the patient how head and eye movements can compensate.[15] Progress the patient as follows:[15]
   a. movements leading the eye from attended to unattended space
   b. eye movements into the unattended space
   c. eye movements without the use of head movements
   d. incorporate the patient's increased awareness and scanning into more difficult visual perceptual and visual motor tasks
4. Place all necessary items for functional independence within the patient's field of vision.[49]

References

1. Cohen AH, Rein LD. The effect of head trauma on the visual system: The doctor of optometry as a member of the rehabilitation team. *J Amer Optometric Association.* 1992;63(8):530-536.
2. Warren M. *Visuo Spatial Skills: Assessment and Intervention Strategies.* AOTA Self Study Series: *Cognitive Rehabilitation.* The American Occupational Therapy Association; 1994.
3. Hellerstein L, Freed S. Rehabilitative optometric management of a traumatic brain injury patient. *J of Behavioral Optometry.* 1994;5(6):143-147.

4. Falk NS, Askionoff EB. The primary care optometric evaluation of the traumatic brain injury patient. *J Amer Optometric Association.* 1992;63(8):547-553.
5. Gianutsos R, Perlin R, Mazerolle KA, et al. Rehabilitation optometric services for persons emerging from coma. *J Head Trauma Rehabil.* 1989;4(2):17-25.
6. Padula WV, Argyris S, Ray J. Visual evoked potentials: Evaluating treatment for post-trauma vision syndrome in patients with traumatic brain injuries. *Brain Injury.* 1994; 8(2):125-133.
7. Padula WV, Shapiro J. Post-traumatic vision syndrome caused by head injury. In: Padula WV (ed.). *A Behavioral Vision Approach For Persons with Physical Disabilities.* Santa Ana, Optometric Extension Program Foundation, Inc.; 1988.
8. Post RB, Leibowitz HW. Two modes of processing visual information: Implications for assessing visual impairment. *American Journal of Optometry and Physiological Optics.* 1986;63:94-96.
9. Warren M. Providing low vision rehabilitation services with occupational therapy and ophthalmology: A program description. *Amer J Occup Ther.* Oct 1995;49(9):877-883.
10. Vogel MS. An overview of head trauma for the primary care practitioner: Part II-Ocular damage associated with head trauma. *J Amer Optometric Assoc.* 1992;63:542-546.
11. Zoltan B. Visual, visual perceptual and perceptual-motor deficits in brain injured adults: Evaluation, treatment and functional implications. In: Kraft GH, Berrol S (eds.). *Physical Medicine and Rehabilitation Clinics of North America.* Philadelphia, WB Saunders Co.; 1992.
12. Zoltan B, Ryckman D. Head injury in adults. In: Pedretti L (ed.). *Occupational Therapy for Physical Dysfunction* (2nd edition). St. Louis, CV Mosby; 1985.
13. Gianutsos R, Matheson P. The rehabilitation of visual perceptual disorders attributable to brain injury. In: Meir MJ, Benton AL, Diller L (eds.). *Neuropsychological Rehabilitation.* New York, Guilford University Press; 1987.
14. Watson GR, Whittaker S, Steciw M. *Pepper Visual Skills for Reading Test* (2nd ed.). Lilburn, GA, Bear Consultants, Inc.; 1995.
15. Bouska MJ, Kauffman NA, Marcus SE. Disorders of the visual perceptual system. In: Umphred DA (ed). *Neurological Rehabilitation* (2nd ed). St. Louis, CV Mosby; 1990.
16. Beaver KA, Mann WC. Overview of technology for low vision. *Amer J Occup Ther.* Oct 1995;49(9):913-921.
17. Lampert J, Lapolice DJ. Functional considerations in evaluation and treatment of the client with low vision. *Amer J Occup Ther.* Oct 1995;49(9):885-890.
18. Vezzetti D. Capacity, content, control: A model for analyzing the cognitive demands of activity. *Occup Ther Pract.* 1989;1(1):9-17.
19. Neger RE. The evaluation of diplopia in head trauma. *J Head Trauma Rehabil.* 1989;4(2):27-34.
20. Zihl J. Cerebral disturbances of elementary visual functions. In: Brown JW (ed.). *Neuropsychology of Visual Perception.* New Jersey, Lawrence Erlbaum Assoc.; 1989.
21. Macdonald J. An investigation of body scheme in adults with cerebral vascular accident. *Am J Occup Ther.* 1960;14:72-79.
22. Malec J. Training the brain-injured client in behavioral self-management skills. In: Edelstein BA and Couture ET (eds). *Behavioral Assessment and Rehabilitation of the Traumatically Brain-Damaged.* New York, Plenum Press; 1984.
23. Parker RS. *Traumatic Brain Injury and Neuropsychological Impairment.* New York, Springer-Verlag; 1990.
24. Warren M. Including occupational therapy in low vision rehabilitation. *Amer J Occup Ther.* Oct 1995;49(9):857-859.
25. Zoltan B, Jabri J, Panikoff L, and Ryckman D. *Perceptual Motor Evaluation for Head Injured and Other Neurologically Impaired Adults.* San Jose, California. Santa Clara Valley Medical Center, Occupational Therapy Department; 1983.
26. Baillet R, Blood K, Bach-y-Rita P. Visual field rehabilitation in the cortically blind. *J Neurol Neurosurg Psychiat* (to be published).
27. Lieberman S, Cohen AH, Rubin J. NYSOA K-D test. *J Am Optom Assoc.* 1983;54(7):631-637.
28. Gordon WA, Ruckdeschel Hibbard M, Egelko S, et al. Perceptual remediation in patients with right brain damage: A comprehensive program. *Arch Phys Med Rehabil.* June 1985;66:353-359.

29. Diller L, Gordon W. Interventions for cognitive deficits in brain-injured adults. *J Consult Clin Psychol.* 1981;49(6):822-834.

30. Piasetsky E, Ben-Yishay Y, Weinberg J. The systematic remediation of specific disorders: Selected application of methods derived in a clinical research setting. In: Trexler LE (ed.). *Cognitive Rehabilitation Conceptualization and Intervention.* New York, Plenum Press; 1982.

31. Cook EA, Luschen L, Sikes S. Dressing training for an elderly woman with cognitive and perceptual impairments. *Amer J Occup Ther.* July 1991;45(7):652-654.

32. Cohen M, GrossWasser Z, Banchadske R, Appel A. Convergence insufficiency in brain-injured patients, *Brain Injury.* 1989;3(2):187-191.

33. Anton HA, Hershler C, Lloyd P, Murray D. Visual neglect and extinction: A new test. *Arch Phys Med Rehabil;* 1988;69:1013-1016.

34. Butters CM, Kirsch NL, Reeves G. The effect of lateralized dynamic stimuli on unilateral spatial neglect following right hemisphere lesions. *Neurology and Neuroscience.* 1990;2:39-46.

35. Caplan B. Assessment of unilateral neglect: A new reading test. *J of Clinical and Experimental Neuropsychology.* 1986;(4):359-364.

36. Caplan B. Stimulus affects in unilateral neglect? *Cortex.* 1985;21:69-89.

37. Ferro JM, Kertesz A, and Black SE. Subcortical Neglect. *Neurology.* 1987;37:1487-1492.

38. Baynes K, Holtzman JD, Volpe BT. Components of visual attention: Alterations in response pattern to visual stimuli following parietal lobe infarction. *Brain.* 1986:99-114.

39. Calvanio, Petrone PN, Levine D. Left visual spatial neglect is both environment-centered and body-centered. *Neurology.* 1987;37:1179-1183.

40. Riddoch MJ, Humphreys GW. Perceptual and action systems in unilateral visual neglect. In: Jeannerod, M (ed). *Neurophysiological and Neuropsychological Aspects of Spatial Neglect.* New York, North-Holland; 1987.

41. Cabay M, King LJ. Sensory integration and perception: The foundation for concept formation. *Occup Ther Pract.* 1989;1(1):18-27.

42. Wilson B, Cockburn J, Halligan P. Development of a behavioral test of visuospatial neglect. *Arch Phys Med Rehabiol.* Feb 1987;68:98-102.

43. Wilson B, Cockburn J, Baddely A. *The Behavioral Inattention Test.* Bury St. Edmunds, Thames Valley Test Co.; 1987.

44. Hartman-Maeir A, Katz N. Validity of the Behavioral Inattention Test (BIT): Relationships with functional tasks. *Amer J Occup Ther.* June 1995;49(6):507-516.

45. Zoltan B. Remediation of visual-perceptual and perceptual-motor deficits. In: Rosenthal M, Griffith ER, Bond MR and Miller JD (eds.). *Rehabilitation of the Adult and Child with Traumatic Brain Injury.* Philadelphia, FA Davis Co.; 1990.

46. Rossi PW, Kheyfets S, Reding MJ. Fresnel prisms improve visual perception in stroke patients with homonomous hemianopia or unilateral visual neglect. *Neurology.* 1990;40:1597-1599.

47. Butters CM, Kirsch N. Combined and separate effects of eye patching and visual stimulation on unilateral neglect following stroke. *Arch Phys. Med Rehabil.* 1990;73:1133-1138.

48. Dick RJ, Wood RG, Bradshaw JL, Bradshaw JA. Programmable visual display for diagnosing, assessing and rehabilitating unilateral neglect. *Med and Biol Eng and Comput.* 1987;25:109-111.

49. Van Deusen J. Unilateral neglect: Suggestions for research by occupational therapists. *Amer J Occup Ther.* 1988;42(7):441-446.

CHAPTER 4

Apraxia

Apraxia is the inability to perform certain skilled purposeful movements in the absence of loss of motor power, sensation or coordination. Although the conceptualization of apraxia as a motor programming disorder has been universally accepted, the exact nature of the programming deficit has remained controversial.[1-5] Heilman and Rothi envision a model of motor planning in which there are visuokinesthetic motor engrams which are stored in the left parietal lobe.[3] Information from this area then activates the pre-motor cortex in the left and then the right hemispheres through the corpus callosum. Building on these concepts, some studies have provided evidence that apraxia may result "from lesions disconnecting the areas where stimuli instigating the movement are processed from the center, where the plan of action must be evoked and programmed, in order to activate the motor cortex neurons."[6]

Many theorize that apraxia is a disturbance to a complex functional system involving two basic functional processes, ie, planning and execution.[7] Roy and Square elaborate on this assumption in their belief that there are two systems which allow us to act in the world: conceptual and production.[4] The conceptual system incorporates three types of knowledge relative to motor planning. These categories of knowledge include knowledge of objects and tools in terms of the action and function they serve, knowledge of actions independent of tools or objects but into which tools or objects may be incorporated, and knowledge relevant to the seriation of single actions into a sequence. In addition to this internal knowledge, perceptual and contextual information provide the individual with an "externalization" of knowledge about the function of the conceptualization of action. The first component is focused on the object or tool which is to be used for a particular function. The next component focuses on the actions performed in carrying out these functions. Perceptual abilities come into play next in selecting an object to perform an action. For example, if the appropriate object is not nearby, the individual may use an object or tool which shares the same characteristics or attributes with the appropriate one.

The second, or production, system of motor action is hypothesized to consist of a number of parallel systems which may operate somewhat independently.[4] Control may shift from one level to another with performance of action involved with a delicate balance between higher and lower level processes. Higher level processes demand attention and keep the action sequence directed toward the intended goal. The lower level system is more autonomous, and involves action programs which require minimal attention demands and " ...which adaptations to environmental constraints are made through existing neural networks."[4]

Apraxia can be a problem in the production system through a temporal-spatial disorder or a disruption to fine motor control. Errors in motor sequencing can occur as a result of damage to either hemisphere.[8] Depending on the location of damage, the type of motor planning deficit which can occur will change. Deficits associated with right brain damage, for example, include difficulties with visual synthesis and analysis for interpreting imitation, commands, spatial organization and spatial thinking for movement production, and unilateral inattention for the interpretation of imitation and production of movements.[5] Apraxia is commonly seen with aphasia, but aphasia does occur without apraxia. Some hypothesize that praxis and language use two different but partly overlapping networks.[9]

When evaluating the apraxic patient, it must be determined which part or parts of the processing system is impaired.[10] Research has shown "...the functional systems and the neural systems of praxis for various parts of the body are sufficiently different that composite measures of praxis probably have no meaning."[11] A comprehensive evaluation, therefore, requires the inclusion of items testing motor planning with specific body parts. Recent research also indicates a performance difference in patients between less representational acts and more representational acts, as well as improvement of performance on imitation. Apraxia evaluation has also recently expanded and is no longer limited to gestural production. It now includes the evaluation of the patient's ability to recognize and discriminate gestures.[5] The therapist must also differentiate between the patient's ability to perform transitive movements (those directed at object manipulation) and intransitive movements (those meant to express ideas or feelings).[6]

In summary, apraxia may take several different forms, with a breakdown occurring in the conceptual and/or production systems. The deficit may be associated with spatiotemporal, temporal or memory activated problems. The major types of apraxia include ideomotor, ideational, oral, constructional and dressing apraxia. The definition, evaluation and treatment of these categories of deficits are described in the following sections.

Ideomotor Apraxia

Ideomotor apraxia is the inability to imitate gestures or perform a purposeful motor task on command even though the patient fully understands the idea or concept of the task.[12,13] These patients, although unable to perform on command, retain kinesthetic memory patterns and the ability to carry out many old habitual motor tasks automatically.[14] Often associated with left hemisphere damage, ideomotor apraxia is hypothesized by some to take two forms.[2,3] The first form is the result of lesions or trauma where visuo-kinesthetic motor engrams are stored. The second form is related to damage to the areas where the engrams are connected to the motor area of the frontal lobes. Clinically, damage to either area will result in the patient having trouble performing movements on command. Patients with "disconnection" lesions where the engrams remain intact, however, should be able to discriminate between poor and correct task performance.[15]

Ideomotor apraxia is a multi-dimensional disorder involving different sensory motor connections.[16] It involves the modality of elicitation, different motor programs which relate to the body part utilized, different conceptual representations or levels of meaningfulness, and "different anatomies for the various interactions of body part and modality."[16] All these dimensions must be included in any comprehensive evaluation of ideomotor apraxia. Performance should be assessed at the command, imitation and real object level. The patient's ability to motor plan utilizing different body parts such as buccofacial, limb and total body movements is also important information.

It has also been found that intransitive movements, or those movements which convey ideas or feelings, are good measures of ideomotor apraxia.[6] These movements relate to a repertoire of motor acts that are well practiced. In addition, they can be designated with a verbal label and have a definite conformation. This allows for easy comparison against the established standard.

One final consideration in the evaluation of ideomotor apraxia is the need for a qualitative analysis of the patient's performance. The patient with ideomotor apraxia will exhibit common errors in motor performance. These errors are outlined as follows:[17]

1. Body parts as objects
2. Altered proximity
3. Altered plane
4. Fragmentary responses
5. Poor distal differentiation
6. Gestural enhancement
7. Vocal overflow
8. Perseveration
9. Manipulation of body part

Functionally, ideomotor apraxia is considered to be less severe than the related deficit of ideational apraxia.[13] The patient with ideomotor apraxia is unable to perform skilled movements on command, but improves with imitation and further improves with the use of the actual object.[6,16] Research has also indicated that these patients improve in certain aspects of their movements when visual and somaesthetic cues are provided.[1]

Ideational Apraxia

The concept of ideational apraxia as a separate entity from ideomotor apraxia has been somewhat controversial.[6] The majority of theorists, researchers and clinicians believe the two can be differentiated. Ideational apraxia is a disability in carrying out complex sequential motor acts, which is caused by a disruption of the conception, rather than the execution, of the motor act.[12,17,18] It is a loss of knowledge of tool function. The errors of the ideational apraxic patient generally occur not from the utilization of single objects in isolation, but in planning more complex events.[17]

The mental process for conceptual sequencing that allows one to relate the symbolism of object names and visual imagery to a related motor performance is lost.[19] Frequently complex acts cannot be performed, whereas simple isolated acts or parts of acts remain. In responding to a command, the more hypothetical the request, the more difficulty the patient has.[19] He cannot pretend to perform an act or describe the function of an object. For example, if given a cigarette and a match and told to light the cigarette, the patient may put the match in his mouth or put the unlighted match to the cigarette. He also cannot describe the match's function.

Ideational apraxia always affects performance bilaterally.[17] There should be no significant difference between right and left hand performance beyond that expected from natural hand preference. As with the patient with ideomotor apraxia, there should be a qualitative assessment of the patient's motor performance. Common errors which characterize performance include:[17]

1.   Elements occur in the wrong order. The person might pour water in the cup before putting tea in.
2.   Sections of the sequence are omitted. The kettle is put on the stove with no water inside.
3.   Two or more elements may be blended together. The person lifts sugar toward the cup, while at the same time making a stirring motion.
4.   The action remains incomplete. Cutting their meat, such people take one slice at it and try to eat it, even though it has not been completely cut.
5.   The action overshoots what is necessary. Asked to take off his coat, the person proceeds to take off all his clothes. Instead of a drop of milk in the cup for the tea, he will fill the whole cup.
6.   Objects are used inappropriately, either for the context, or overall. Instead of spooning sugar into the cup of tea, the person eats the sugar from the spoon. A pencil might be used as a comb. The candle is struck instead of the match.
7.   Movements may be made in the wrong plane or wrong direction. The person might "stir" his tea by lifting the spoon up and down. He might make a pulling-away motion when trying to push in a plug.
8.   Many of these errors can be interpreted as perseveratory. After pouring the tea from the pot into the cup, the person might then perform a similar act with the sugar bowl, instead of spooning it in.
9.   Many patients, in their endeavors to testify what they realize is wrong, may make several abortive runs at a task before succeeding or becoming frustrated and giving up.

Infrequently, the ideational or conceptual objective of a motor performance is lost, while the motor performance remains intact because the motor sequence belongs to the intact hemisphere, whereas the ideational sequence is found in the damaged hemisphere. Denny-Brown[20] refers to this syndrome as adextrous apraxia. For example, a left-handed man has learned to write with his right hand. After a right-sided brain lesion, he is unable to conceptualize and form an intelligible work; however, he retains the skill to form written letters with his right hand.[20]

Evaluation of Ideomotor and Ideational Apraxia

As previously described, these apraxias are very similar and difficult to differentiate. The test is the same for them; only the quality of the response varies slightly. When asked to do a task, a person with motor or ideomotor apraxia would not be able to do it on command, but could do it automatically at the appropriate time. A person with ideational apraxia could not do it even automatically, although he has the motor capacity to do it.

TEST 1: THE SOLET TEST FOR APRAXIA[21]*

Description:
This is a 40-item evaluation technique designed to further professional understanding of apraxia itself, as well as for use in treatment planning. It identifies two variations of apraxia—ideational and ideomotor—by differentiating the level of concreteness of impaired actions. Gestures, object use, demonstration of use of missing object, and nonrepresentational movements are included. Commands are presented to distinguish three areas of possible body part involvement: buccal-facial, right or left (or both) upper extremities, and the whole body. The ability to follow verbal directions, to select described actions from a series of demonstrations, and to imitate the examiner are evaluated.

Scoring:
Nonstandardized. The test supplies a structure for detailed examination of the actual individual client's apraxic response, rather than only indicating intact or impaired praxis. Response characteristics discussed include groping and hesitation, improvement on imitations, and displaced plane of movement. The test is followed by a series of treatment implications.
To improve validity, rule out incomprehension of the directions, paralysis or paresis of the affected side.

TEST 2: PRAXIS TEST—SANTA CLARA VALLEY MEDICAL CENTER[22]†

Description:
This is a ten-item test, which is administered to command, involving both imitation and real objects (items 1 to 5 only). Items include buccal-facial, unilateral and bilateral limb, and total body tasks.

Scoring:
Severely impaired—action is almost unrecognizable.
Impaired—action is carried out imperfectly (eg, directional problems, hesitation) or with some delay.
Intact—action is carried out immediately and correctly.
To improve validity, rule out paresis of affected side, incoordination, unilateral neglect, and incomprehension of directions.

Reliability:
Inter-rater reliability ($r = 0.99$) was established for this test with a sample of adult patients with head trauma.[30]
In addition, inter-item correlations indicated a high degree of correlation between several test items (see Appendix A). Additional research should indicate whether administering all test items is unnecessary duplication.

TEST 3: PRAXIS SUBTEST OF THE L.O.T.C.A.[25]

Description:
The praxis subtest of the L.O.T.C.A. contains three parts: motor imitation, utilization of objects, and symbolic actions.

Scoring:
1 point—patient is unable to produce any task

---

*The Solet Test for Apraxia is available through its author: Jo M. Solet, MOT, OTR, 5 Channing Road, Newton Center, MA, 02159.

---

†Reproduced with permission from Santa Clara Valley Medical Center, San Jose, CA.

2 points—patient is only able to imitate movements
3 points—patient is able to imitate movements and to manipulate with objects
4 points—patient performs all tasks.

Reliability:
Inter-rater reliability with Spearman's rank correlation coefficient between raters ranged from .82 to .97 for the various subtests.

Validity:
Wilcoxin's two-sample test was used to compare each patient group with the control group. Tests differentiated at the .001 level of significance between the control group and each of the patient groups.

Treatment for Ideomotor and Ideational Apraxia

Utilizing a Remedial Approach:

1. Provide proprioceptive, tactile, and kinesthetic input prior to and during a task. For example, take the patient's leg through the required motion to propel his wheelchair.
2. Apply concepts from the Affolter approach: place your hand over the hand of the patient and guide him through the required task. For example, during hygiene activities, if the patient used his toothbrush on his hair, do not verbally cue him that he has made a mistake. Guide his hand with the toothbrush, without verbalizations, away from his hair and into his mouth or down to the faucet in an appropriate sequence (Bonfils, personal communication). Frequently, this will elicit recognition on the patient's part and he may be able to take over the normal sequence of movement. "Guiding can be a way of respectfully communicating by stopping one engram, and, replacing it with another without words" (Bonfils, personal communication).

Utilizing an Adaptive Approach:

1. Keep verbal commands to a minimum, and place activity on a subcortical level. For example, instead of the verbal command, "Lock your brakes," say to the patient, "There's something on your brakes."
2. Identify specifically the type of apraxia that is present, eg, unilateral limb, total body. Are movements away from the body or toward the body affected? Use this information in your treatment approach. For instance, the patient with unilateral or bilateral limb apraxia will do better with gross motor, total body activities and will do worse if activities are broken down into segments. For example, in coming to standing, giving directions and breaking down the activity into segments such as scooting, pushing, and leaning, will only serve to confuse the patient. A simple command, such as "Get up," puts the activity on a more automatic total body level.
3. Activities should be performed in as nearly normal an environment as possible. For example, dressing should be done in the morning at the bedside instead of in the clinic in the middle of the day. If possible, cooking activities should be done in the home, or at least with familiar utensils.

4. Have the patient close his eyes and visualize the required movements before attempting to carry them out.
5. Provide support to the patient when he becomes frustrated. Explain to him that you know that he is not being uncooperative and that certain movements are difficult for him. Provide some activities during therapy that will assure the patient success.
6. Educate the patient and his family about the apraxia. Areas where safety is an issue should be highlighted.

Oral Apraxia

Oral apraxia is the difficulty in forming and organizing intelligible words, although the musculature required to do so remains intact. This differs from dysarthria, in which the muscles are affected and the speech is slurred. These patients may be able to use the tongue for automatic acts such as chewing and swallowing, but may not be able to stick it out when asked. Some believe oral apraxia is a disorder of the linguistic-conceptual system.[26-28] The wrong movement is selected for execution at the highest level of programming the motoric act. Others believe it is a problem with the production system. Roy and Square believe both systems are involved and state oral apraxia "involves both top-down and bottom-up influences which operate in parallel."[27]

Evaluation and Treatment for Oral Apraxia

Evaluation and treatment for oral apraxia are usually done by the speech pathologist. However, if there is no speech pathologist available, a simple screening test can be used. First, ask the patient to lick his lips. If he cannot do so on command, put some honey or peanut butter on his lips and observe whether he automatically licks it off. If he can lick his lips automatically but not on command, he is probably apraxic. If he cannot lick them at all he is probably dysarthric. Some of the evaluations previously described in the ideomotor/ideational section also contain items which test for oral apraxia.

Constructional Apraxia

Constructional apraxia is the impairment in producing designs in two or three dimensions, by copying, drawing, or constructing, whether upon command or spontaneously.[29,30] Constructional apraxia results from lesions in either cerebral hemisphere and limits the patient's ability to perform purposeful acts while using objects in his environment.[31]

A controversy exists about the occurrence of constructional apraxia among patients with right- and left-sided brain damage. It is widely believed that patients with right-sided damage show a greater incidence of the deficit.[32] However, others hypothesize an equal distribution of the symptoms of both right and left groups.[33] The authors hypothesizing an equal distribution of symptoms in both groups insist that aphasic patients often have the deficit but are not included in test groups for patients with left-sided brain damage, since they are frequently either confused or unable to understand directions.

Although patients with both right and left hemiplegia display this deficit, a distinct difference between the two groups, supported more by observation of quality of response than by objective perceptual testing,[34] has been widely described in the literature. It seems apractic patients with right-sided lesions, with or without visual field deficits, are characterized by a visual-spatial disability, such that they lack perspective, the exact location of a figure in space, and the ability to analyze parts in relation to each other.[35-38] Apractic patients with left-sided lesions have spatial problems only if a visual field deficit exists simultaneously, but overall exhibit an executive or planning problem.[35,37,39,40] Thus, these patients, regardless of whether they are able to see things in correct perspective, have trouble in initiating a planned sequence of movements when trying to construct an object.

Patients with right-sided cerebral damage tend to be less hesitant in their drawings and use a piecemeal approach rather than an orderly one.[39] They frequently draw on the diagonal, neglect the left side of the drawing, and have no particular way for using the space on the page.[37] Their designs are often very complex, often unrecognizable, but do include many pieces of the drawing scattered with proper spatial relationships to one another.[41-43] Frequently, lines in the drawing are overscored in an attempt to correct or finish the task.[39] Their drawings show that they have a great deal of difficulty with perspective, and constructing anything with three dimensions, such as blocks or bricks, is extremely difficult.[30] These patients are usually not helped by the presence of a model, and when given some landmarks, eg, part of the drawing filled in, their work is unaffected or they are made more confused.[37,42] Short-term visual memory is hypothesized to be poor and the patient seems unable to keep the model in mind. After several trials at a particular task, no learning appears to take place.[42,44]

On the other hand, patients with left-sided damage tend to be very hesitant in their task and produce designs of great simplicity.[45] They often cannot draw angles, their designs are poor in outline and they have apparent difficulty in execution.[39] These patients seem to have more general intellectual impairment, and it is thought that their ability to establish the program task is lost or diminished.[42,46] However, their performance is often facilitated by the presence of a model, and often they tend to move closer and closer to it (called the closing-in effect by Mayer-Gross[47]) until finally their copy is superimposed on the model.[37] Landmarks, ie, part of the picture filled in, appear helpful.[42] After several trials, these patients seem to learn the task and can repeat it more easily.[42] Memories for visual and auditory images are thought to be short, thus drawing to command or from memory is affected more than copying a model.

Functionally, constructional apraxia has been related to body scheme problems, dressing apraxia and meal preparation.[48-52] In a study of fifty-four head injured patients, Neidstat found a significant correlation between constructional praxis and meal preparation. Neidstat concludes that constructional abilities may contribute to meal preparation performance and believes it is "...functionally relevant for rehabilitation specialists to use block design type tests to evaluate the constructional skills of the clients who have brain injury."[53] In a study of one hundred and one C.V.A. patients, Warren found that disorders of body scheme and constructional apraxia jointly contributed to the presence of dressing apraxia.[51]

Lorenze and Cancro,[54] using the WAIS block design and object assembly subtests, found that patients who did poorly on these tests did not acquire dressing and grooming skills even after practice in dressing. In patients with right-sided lesions, the presence of severe constructional apraxia with perceptual problems has been found to relate to the same lack of independence in daily living skills.[55]

Historically, occupational therapists have used primarily a remedial approach to treat constructional apraxia.[53] The effectiveness of this approach, however, has come into question. In a study of 45 adult male head injured patients, both a remedial and adaptive treatment approach were given. The subject group which received the remedial approach received training in parquetry block designs. The group receiving the adaptive approach received training in food preparation. The results of the study indicated that they had task specific learning. In other words, the parquetry group did better on post-test on parquetry tasks, and the functional group performed better on the specific functional task on post-test. There was no transfer of learning to other functional or constructional tasks or activities. This important study suggests two possible directions in treatment decision making. First, for transfer of learning to occur, training must occur in a variety of environments using targeted strategies for task completion.[56] Secondly, since learning appears to be task specific, an adaptive functional approach would have more impact than a remedial approach.

Evaluation for Constructional Apraxia

TEST 1: COPYING DESIGNS—TWO DIMENSIONAL

Description:
The therapist hands the patient paper and pencil and asks him to copy the design on the stimulus card. A separate sheet of paper is used to copy each stimulus card. There are several variations on this test, none of them standardized. For example:
- Copy a previously drawn line drawing of a house (Figure 4-1), a flower, and a clock face.[57]
- Copy geometric designs (Figure 4-2).

Scoring:
Nonstandardized.
Each drawing is scored on a scale of 1 to 3.
Score 1 if the drawing is essentially correct, no lines are omitted or added, and spatial arrangement is correct.
Score 2 if the drawing is partially defective owing to omissions of some lines, rotations or disproportions between single parts, but not to such an extent as to prevent identification of the figure.
Score 3 if the drawing is unrecognizable.
Intact—scores of drawings mostly 1
Impaired—scores of drawings mostly 2
Severe—scores of drawings mostly 3
To improve validity, rule out incoordination, especially if the patient is using his nondominant hand (unilateral neglect). Right and left hemiplegics have qualitative differences in their drawings (see description of deficit).

TEST 2: GRAPHIC DESIGNS—SANTA CLARA VALLEY MEDICAL CENTER[22]

Description:
The patient is asked to copy from prepared cards each of the following: horizontal line, vertical line, cross, circle, square, triangle, diamond, cube, house and clock.

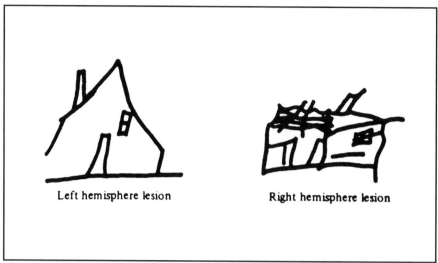

Figure 4-1. Example of impaired performance in drawing a house.

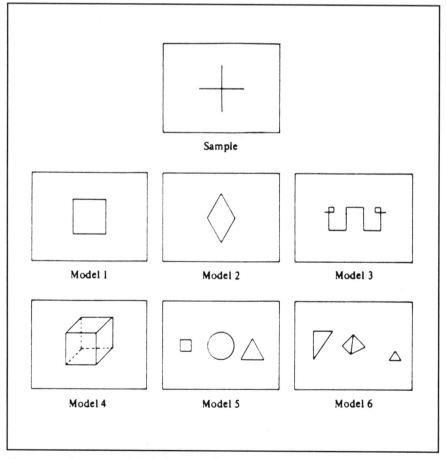

Figure 4-2. Copy geometric designs test.[54]

Scoring:
Severely impaired—design is almost totally unrecognizable
Impaired—design lacks perspective, is rotated or partially unrecognizable
Intact—design is copied accurately
To improve validity, rule out incoordination, unilateral neglect, visual field cuts, and other visual problems.

Reliability:
Inter-rater reliability (r = 0.98) was established for this test in a study of adult patients who sustained head trauma.[23] In the same study, frequency data indicated no variance in performance for copying horizontal and vertical lines, a cross, a square, and a triangle. All other items appeared to be good discriminators of dysfunction.

TEST 3: MATCHSTICK DESIGNS[55]

Description:
The therapist makes a design using matchsticks and asks the patient to copy it. The designs should vary in complexity, from using two to nine wooden kitchen matches. There is no standardized form of this test. The therapist makes up the designs.

Scoring:
Subjective.
Intact—patient copies all designs correctly within a reasonable length of time.
To improve validity, rule out unilateral neglect, motor apraxias.

Reliability:
A refined matchstick design test[22] was utilized as part of a constructional praxis subtest in a study of adult patients with head trauma.[23] Intertest correlations showed the correlation between the matchstick and block design tests to be extremely high (r=0.92). This high correlation (r=0.9222) had also been found in a study conducted by Baum and Hall.[48] This combined research indicates that administering both a matchstick design and a block design test is unnecessary duplication. In addition, item analysis revealed a higher overall reliability when the matchstick design test was deleted rather than the block design test. It is therefore recommended that a matchstick design test be utilized only if a block design test if unavailable.

TEST 4: BLOCK DESIGN, SANTA CLARA VALLEY MEDICAL CENTER[58]

Description:
The patient is asked to duplicate block designs from prepared models.

Scoring:
Severely impaired—design is almost totally unrecognizable
Intact—design is copied accurately
To improve validity, rule out motor apraxias.

Reliability:
Inter-rater reliability (r = 0.96) was established for this test in a study of adult head trauma patients.[23] In addition, item analysis indicated a high degree of test reliability (alpha = 0.87) for this test given in conjunction with the Santa Clara Valley Medical Center graphic design test.[23]

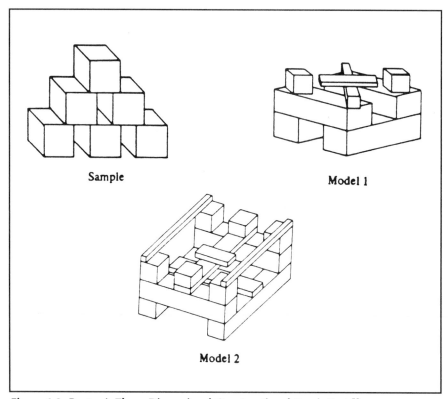

Sample

Model 1

Model 2

Figure 4-3. Benton's Three-Dimensional Constructional Praxis Test.[59]

TEST 5: BENTON'S THREE-DIMENSIONAL CONSTRUCTIONAL PRAXIS TEST[59,60]

Description:
The patient is asked to copy block constructions composed of blocks of various sizes (Figure 4-3). The test set of 29 blocks is organized in a shallow box (Figure 4-4) and placed on the patient's unaffected side. The sample is placed in front of the patient and he is told to copy it. The therapist demonstrates first and then returns the blocks to the box. The patient then tries to copy the model. If he is successful, the blocks are returned to the box and the first test model is placed in front of him at a 45 degree angle. The blocks of all the models are glued together for easy handling. The patient is given five minutes to copy the model. Then the blocks are returned to the box and the procedure is repeated for the second test model.

Scoring:
Nonstandardized.
Each block is scored one point if correct and zero points if incorrect according to whether is was:
Omitted—the block not included in the construction
Substituted—the patient substituted a block of a different size from the one in the model
Displaced—the block placed on the wrong corner or section of the figure.
(Blocks that were correctly placed but not exactly lined up with those immediately above or below them, eg, slightly rotated, are considered correct. Scoring is done in layers, from the bottom layer up, and blocks are scored in relation to those below it.)
Intact—score of 22-23 (90 percent of normal controls).

Apraxia   **65**

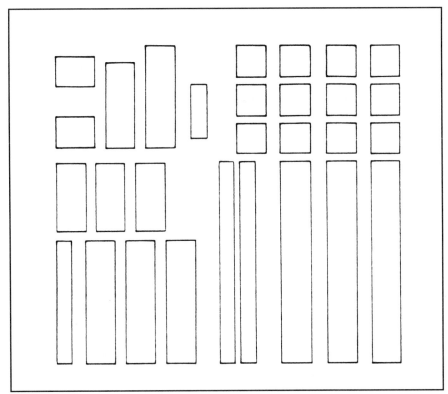

Figure 4-4. Arrangement of blocks for the three-dimensional constructional praxis test.

Impaired—score of 20-21 (9 percent of control group).
Severe—score of 19 or below (1 percent of control group).[61]
To improve validity, rule out motor apraxias.

TEST 6: THE BENDER-GESTALT TEST[62]

Description:
The patient is given a blank piece of paper and a pencil. He is shown nine cards, one at a time, and asked to draw the design he sees on the card. He draws all nine designs on one piece of paper.

Scoring:
Standardized.
In testing its reliability, the authors report a test-retest correlation of $r = 0.71$ and a score reliability of $r = 0.90$. This test has elaborate directions for scoring. To learn how to score it, one must consult the manual. However, one can make observations from the results even if it is not scored.
To improve validity, rule out unilateral neglect, hemianopsia, poor eyesight, poor coordination due to paresis, or use of nondominant hand.

OTHER TESTS

Almost any constructional task can be utilized as a constructional praxis evaluation; some of them have been described elsewhere in this chapter, so we will only list some of the more common ones here: copying pegboard designs, puzzles, copying block designs similar to designs on the Sechsler Adult Intelligence Scale, Draw-A-Man Test, Frostig's Spatial Relations Test.

Validity of Constructional Praxis Tests

Benton[59] believes that the various "constructional apraxia" tests are not necessarily testing the same skill. He found that his Visual Retention Test (a test of copying geometric figures) correlated only weakly with his Three-Dimensional Constructional Praxis Test. Pehoski[60] also found only a weak correlation between her copy drawing test and Benton's Three-Dimensional Constructional Praxis Test.

The various tests vary in complexity, in the type of movement and dexterity required to do the task, in the demands of higher intellectual function, and in the involvement of two or three spatial dimensions. For example, the task of copying geometric designs requires more precise graphic movements and a higher degree of sensorimotor integration than block building or matchstick arranging.[59]

Treatment for Constructional Apraxia

Utilizing a Remedial Approach:

1. Have the patient practice various 2-D and 3-D table top activities. Utilize techniques such as backward chaining.[49]
2. Provide tactile and kinesthetic cues to the patient by having the patient explore a 3-D model with his hands before constructing his model.
3. Apply concepts from the Affolter approach by providing tactile kinesthetic guiding to the patient during constructional tasks. For example, if the patient is working on a work related nuts and bolts assembly task, place your hand over the patient's and guide him through the necessary sequence. Reduce or remove guiding as the patient takes over the task.

Utilizing an Adaptive Approach:

1. Identify performance components which are impaired as the result of constructional apraxia, ie, meal preparation, vocational tasks. Provide assistive techniques during the task such as backward chaining.[49] Present a partially completed task and ask the patient to complete it. For example, placing the knife and glass and partially completed place setting.[49]
2. Apply concepts from the Dynamic Interactional Approach: identify what task characteristics can be altered to improve performance. For example, the patient may be able to perform assembly tasks if the pieces are laid out in a specific order, or marked with sequential numbers for assembly.
3. Educate the patient and his family about his constructional deficits and how it will affect function. Areas where safety is an issue should be highlighted.

Dressing Apraxia

Dressing apraxia is the inability to dress oneself because of a disorder in body scheme and/or spatial relations. This apraxia is related more to body scheme and spatial deficits than to a difficulty in the motor performance of dressing.[20] The patient makes mistakes of orientation in putting the clothes on backwards, upside-down, or inside-out. Often the patients with right-sided lesions will neglect to dress the left side of the body or put both legs in the same pant leg. Pehoski provides us with the following example of the patient with dressing apraxia.[60]

1. The subject was unable to find the correct sleeve. He looked at the shirt in a puzzled manner and finally put his involved arm into a sleeve, but it was the wrong sleeve.

2. He then had some difficulty getting the sleeve up the involved extremity, but he finally managed to slide it past the elbow and onto the involved shoulder.

3. He then reached around his back as a normal response to find the other sleeve. Since the correct sleeve had not been used at the beginning, the second arm hole was not in back as it should have been, but remained in front. He then came back to the material in front of him and found the second arm hole and put his uninvolved extremity in. The shirt was then on as if it were to be buttoned down the back. He looked puzzled for a moment and then put the material that was in front over his head to the back. Now he had the bulk of the material behind his neck with the two shirt tails hanging over his shoulder in front. Feeling at the back of his neck, he asked, "Where is the collar?" After several seconds of fumbling for the collar and trying to pull the shirt down, he said, "I've fouled up somewhere along the line. The collar is nowhere." (Total time: 3 minutes, 34 seconds.)

Evaluation for Dressing Apraxia

The test for this is strictly a functional one, ie, observe the patient during dressing. Does he have trouble in deciding where to begin or where to find the right armhole? Does he neglect to dress the left half of his body (indication of unilateral neglect)? Does he put the shirt on inside-out or backwards? Does he button it so the buttons are not aligned correctly? All these are signs of dressing apraxia and not just the inability to dress because of motor paralysis. Because there is usually a high degree of correlation between dressing and constructional apraxia, some people have used tests for constructional apraxia to assist in diagnosing or predicting dressing apraxia.[23,54]

Treatment for Dressing Apraxia
Utilizing a Remedial Approach:

1. Apply concepts from the Affolter Approach. The patient is encouraged to start dressing on his own with visual or verbal cues. If the patient does not start dressing, try a verbal cue, "Get dressed please." Then wait to see if the patient is able to recognize the language combined with the visual cue.[63] Provide nonverbal tactile-kinesthetic patient guiding at the beginning and during dressing. As needed, reduce or remove guiding as the patient takes

over the activity. If there is a breakdown in the sequence or the patient is having difficulty, provide guiding again.

2. Apply concepts from the Neurodevelopmental Approach. Provide weight bearing, weight shifting and handling techniques prior to dressing. Set up the activity to "force" the patient to use the affected extremities.

Utilizing an Adaptive Approach:

1. Apply concepts from the Dynamic Interactional Approach. Identify how changing the surface characteristics of dressing can alter performance. For example, does laying one garment at a time versus all clothes at once improve performance? Try dressing training in a variety of ways, ie, sitting on edge of the bed, in wheelchair, etc.

2. Apply concepts from a Functional Adaptive Approach by providing the following to help the patient compensate.
   a. Use labels to distinguish back from front and right from wrong side.
   b. If garment does not have distinguishing labels, the therapist can color code the garment for right-left, back-front, and wrong side-right side.
   c. If patient has trouble matching buttons to the right buttonhole, tell him to start at the bottom of the shirt and find the last button and match it to the last buttonhole. Continue matching upward from there. Or the therapist can color code the bottom button and buttonhole.
   d. Have patient circle the button with his finger to feel that he has it all the way through the buttonhole.

3. Educate the patient and his family regarding his dressing problems and why he is having difficulty. Emphasize that this problem is not related to poor motivation. Train the patient and the family on compensation techniques.

References

1. Clark MA, Merians AS, Kothari A, et al. Spatial planning deficits in limb apraxia. *Brain.* 1994;117:1093-1106.
2. Harrington DL, Haaland KY. Motor sequencing with left hemisphere damage: Are some cognitive deficits specific to limb apraxia? *Brain.* 1992;115:857-874.
3. Heilman KM, Rothi LJG. Apraxia. In: Heilman KM, Valenstein E (eds). *Clinical Neuropsychology.* New York, Oxford University Press; 1985.
4. Roy EA, Square PA. Common considerations in the study of limb, verbal and oral apraxia. In: Roy EA (ed). *Neuropsychological Studies of Apraxia and Related Disorders.* New York, North-Holland; 1985.
5. York CD, Cermak SA. Visual perception and praxis in adults after stroke. *Amer J Occup Ther.* 1995;49(6):543-549.
6. DeRenzi E. Methods of limb apraxia evaluation and their bearing on the interpretation of the disorder. In: EA Roy (ed.) *Neuropsychological Studies of Apraxia and Related Disorders.* New York, North-Holland; 1985.
7. Goodgold-Edwards SA, Cermak S. Integrating motor control and motor learning concepts with neuropsychological perspectives on apraxia and developmental dyspraxia. *Amer J Occup Ther.* 1990;44(5):431-439.
8. Arnadottir G. *The Brain and Behavior: Assessing Cortical Dysfunction Through Activities of Daily Living.* St. Louis, CV Mosby; 1990.

9. Papagno C, Della Sala S, Basso A. Ideomotor apraxia without aphasia and aphasia without apraxia: The anatomical support for a double dissociation. *J Neurol Neurosurg Psychiatry.* 1993;56:286-289.

10. Fraser C, Turton A. The development of the Cambridge apraxia battery. *British J Occupational therapy.* 1986;49,248-252.

11. Barron A, Mattila, WR. Response slowing of older adults: Effects of time limit contingencies on single and dual task performances. *Psychology and Aging.* 1989;4:66-72.

12. Hopkins HL. Occupational therapy management of cerebrovascular accident and hemiplegia. In: Willard H, Spackman C (eds.). *Occupational Therapy* (4th edition). Philadelphia, J.B. Lippincott Company; 1971.

13. Square-Storer P. *Acquired Apraxia of Speech.* New York, Taylor and Francis; 1989.

14. Baillet R, Blood K, Bach-y-Rita P. Visual field rehabilitation in the cortically blind. *J Neurol Neurosurg Psychiat* (to be published).

15. Heilman KM, Rothi LJG, Valenstein E. Two forms of ideomotor apraxia. *Neurology.* 1982;32: 342-346.

16. Baker-Nobles L, Bink MP. Sensory integration in the rehabilitation of blind adults. *Am J Occup Ther.* 1979;33(9):559-564

17. Miller N. *Dyspraxia and its Management.* Gaithersburg, Maryland, Aspen Publications; 1986.

18. Ochipa C, Rothi LJG, Heilman KM. Ideational apraxia: A deficit in tool selection and use. *Ann Neurol.* 1989;25:190-193.

19. Crovitz HF, Harvey MT, Horn RW. Problems in the acquisition of imagery mnemonics: Three brain-damaged cases. *Cortex.* 1979:225-234.

20. Denny-Brown D. The nature of apraxia. *J Nerv Ment Dis.* 1958;126:9-32.

21. Solet JM. Solet test for apraxia. Thesis, Boston University; 1974.

22. Zoltan B, Jabri J, Panikoff L, Ryckman D. *Perceptual Motor Evaluation for Head Injured and Other Neurologically Impaired Adults.* San Jose, California. Santa Clara Valley Medical Center, Occupational Therapy Department; 1983.

23. Baum B. The establishment of reliability and validity of a perceptual evaluation on a sample of adult head trauma patients. Thesis, University of Southern California, December 1981.

24. Fetherlin JM, Kurland L. Self-instruction: A compensatory strategy to increase functional independence with brain-injured adults. *Occup Ther Pract.* 1989;1(1):75-78.

25. Jongbloed L, Stacey S, Brighten C. Stroke rehabilitation: Sensorimotor integrative versus functional treatment. *Amer J Occup Ther.* 1989;43(6):391-397.

26. Berrol S. Issues in cognitive rehabilitation. *Arch Neurol.* Feb 1990;47:219-220.

27. Duchek J. Cognitive dimensions of performance. In: Christiansen C, Baum, C (eds). *Occupational Therapy: Overcoming Human Performance Deficits.* New Jersey, SLACK Inc.; 1991.

28. Stoer P. Chromaticity and achromaticity: Evidence for a functional differentiation in visual field defects. *Brain.* 1987;110:869-886.

29. Cohen RF, Mapou RL. Neuropsychological assessment for treatment planning: A hypothesis-testing approach. *J Head Trauma Rehabil.* March 1988;3(1):12-23.

30. Hecaen H, Penfield W, Bertrand C, Malmo R. The syndrome of apractognosis due to lesions of the minor cerebral hemisphere. *Arch Neurol Psychiat.* 1956;75:400-434.

31. Fahle M. Figure-ground discrimination from temporal information. *Proc R Soc Lond B Biol Sci.* 1993;254(1341):199-203.

32. Fisher B. Effect of trunk control and alignment on limb function. *J Head Trauma Rehabil.* 1987;2(2):72-79.

33. Finlayson MA, Garner SH. *Brain Injury Rehabilitation: Clinical Considerations.* Baltimore, Williams and Wilkins; 1994.

34. Crook T. Psychometric assessment in the elderly. In: Raskin A, Javick L (eds.). *Psychiatric Symptoms and Cognitive Loss in the Elderly.* New York, Hemisphere Publishing Co.; 1979.

35. DeRenzi E, Faglioni P. The relationship between visuo-spatial impairment and construction. *Cortex.* 1967;3:327-342.

36. Gulyas B, Heywood CA, Popplewell DA, Roland PE, Cowey A. Visual form discrimination from color or motion cues: Functional anatomy by positron emission tomography. *Proc. Natl. Acad. Science.* Oct 1994;91:9965-9969.

37. Piercy M, Hecaen H, de Ajuriaguerra J. Constructional apraxia associated with unilateral cerebral lesions: Left and right sided cases compared. *Brain.* 1960;83:225-242.
38. Podolsky S, Schachar R. Clinical manifestations of diabetic retinopathy and other diseases of the eye in the elderly. In: Ordy JM, Bizzee KR (eds.). *Aging. Vol. 10. Sensory Systems and Communication in the Elderly.* New York, Raven Press; 1979.
39. Gainotti G, Tiacci C. Patterns of drawing disability in right and left hemispheric patients. *Neuropsychologia.* 1970;8:379-384.
40. Instructo-Clinic—A Psychophysical Testing Apparatus. Bumpa-Tel, Inc., P.O. Box 611, Cape Cir., Missouri 63701.
41. Glisky E, Schacter D. Remediation of organic memory disorders: Current status and future prospects. *Journal of Head Trauma Rehabilitation.* 1986;1(3):54-63.
42. Hecaen H, Assal G. A comparison of constructive deficits following right and left hemispheric lesions. *Neuropsychologia.* 1970;8:289-303.
43. Kahn HJ, Whitaker HA. Acalculia: An historical review of localization. *Brain and Cogn.* 1991;17:102-1151.
44. Niestadt ME. Occupational therapy treatment for constructional deficits. *Amer J Occup Ther.* 1991;46(2):141-148.
45. McFie J, Zangwill OL. Visual-constructive disabilities associated with lesions of the left cerebral hemisphere. *Brain.* 1960;83:243-259.
46. Doehring DG, Reitan RM, Klove H. Changes in patterns of intelligence test performance associated with homonymous visual field defects. *J Nerv Ment Dis.* 1961;132:227-233.
47. Mayer-Gross W. Some observations of apraxia. *Proc Roy Soc Med.* 1934-1935;28:1203-1212.
48. Baum B, Hall K. Relationship between constructional praxis and dressing in the head injured adult. *Am J Occup Ther.* 1981;35(7):438-442.
49. Bouska MJ, Kauffman NA, Marcus SE. Disorders of the visual perceptual system. In: Umphred DA (ed). *Neurological Rehabilitation (*2nd edition*).* St. Louis, CV Mosby; 1990.
50. Neistadt ME. The relationship between constructional and meal preparation skills. *Arch Phys Med Rehabil.* 1993;74:144-148.
51. Warren M. Relationship of constructional apraxia and body scheme disorders to dressing performance in adult C.V.A. *Amer J Occup Ther.* 1981;35(7):431-437.
52. Williams N. Correlations between copying ability and dressing activities in hemiplegia. *Am J Phys Med.* 1967;46:1332-1340.
53. Neistadt ME. A critical analysis of occupational therapy approach for perceptual deficits in adults with brain injury. *Amer J Occup Ther.* 1990;44:299-304.
54. Lorenze EJ, Cancro R. Dysfunction in visual perception with hemiplegia: its relation to activities of daily livng. *Arch Phys Med.* 1962;43:514-517.
55. Gregory ME, Aitkin JA. Assessment of parietal lobe function in hemiplegia. *Occup Ther.* 1971;34:9-17.
56. Toglia JP. Generalization of treatment: A multicontextual approach to cognitive perceptual impairment in the brain injured adult. *Amer J Occup Ther.* 1991;45(6):505-516.
57. Deitz JC, Tovar VS, Thorn DW, Beeman C. The test of orientation for rehabilitation patients: Interrater reliability. *Amer J Occup Therapy.* 1990;44(9):784-790.
58. Madden DJ. Adult age differences in the time course of visual attention. *Journal of Gerontology.* 1990;45:9-16.
59. Benton AL, Fogel ML. Three-dimensional constructional praxis, a clinical test. *Arch Neurol.* 1962;7:347-354.
60. Pehoski C. Analysis of perceptual dysfunction and dressing in adult hemiplegics. Thesis, Sargent College, Boston University; 1970.
61. Anderson SW, Tranel D. Awareness of disease states following cerebral infarction, dementia, and head trauma: Standardized assessment. *The Clinical Neuropsychologist.* 1989;3(4):327-339.
62. Pascal GK, Suttell B. *The Bender-Gestalt Test—Its Quantification and Validity for Adults.* New York, Grune & Stratton, Inc.; 1951.
63. Bonfils K. Affolter Approach. In: Pedretti L (ed). *Practice Skills for Physical Dysfunction.* St. Louis, CV Mosby; 1995.

CHAPTER 5

Body Scheme Disorders

Body Scheme

An individual's body scheme is a representation of the spatial relations among the parts of the body.[1-4] Through the integration of proprioceptive, tactile and pressure input, the body scheme becomes the "neural foundation for perception of body position and the relationships of the body and its parts."[5] An intact body scheme allows for the spatial indexing of sensory input and is involved in the triggering and guidance of movement.[6] It is the foundation for future skills in environmental perception.[4,7] Sirigi et al hypothesize that there are at least four kinds of representations which contribute to body knowledge processing.[8] These representations are described as follows:[8]

1. The first contains semantic and lexical information about body parts, such as names; the functional relations that exist between body parts, such as the wrist and the ankle (eg, articulations); the functional purpose of the mouth or the ear, etc. These representations are in large part prepositional and are likely to be more strongly linked to the verbal systems.

2. The second contains the category-specific visuospatial representations of an individual's own body, but also of bodies in general. These representations define a structural description of the body and specify in a detailed manner the position of individual parts on the body surface (eg, the nose is in the middle of the face), the proximity relationships that exist *between* body parts (eg, the nose is next to the eyes, the leg is between the ankle and the knee, etc.), and most importantly the *boundaries* that define each body part. These representations are necessary for "part/whole" analysis. They are likely to be more strongly linked to the nonverbal, visual and somatosensory systems.

3. The third level is the emergent body-reference system and is conceptualized as a dynamic, actual body image. It gives information about the position and the changes in position of an individual's own body parts relative to each other and in relation to external space.

4. Motor representations also contribute to the construction of a spatial representation of the body. It is further hypothesized that these components of the body representation system are relatively independent, but can also interact with each other. The degree of interaction depends on the particular task demands.[8]

Since the body scheme has multiple representations, impairment can occur at different levels of body knowledge processing.[1,3,8] Clinically, the patient may exhibit different types of problems. For example, the patient may be able to localize body parts on himself but not on others, or be able to name body parts spatially but not functionally. In addition, the patient's body alignment and positioning may influence the degree of body knowledge.[9] Disturbances in body scheme can include somatognosia, anasognosia, unilateral body neglect, impaired right-left discrimination and finger agnosia. The definition, evaluation and treatment of these disorders are subsequently described. No matter what level or component of body scheme is impaired, associated problems with various self-care activities will be evident.[5]

Somatognosia

Somatognosia, a disturbance in the previously described body scheme, is the lack of awareness of body structure and the failure to recognize one's parts and their relationship to each other. A patient who has such a deficit also has difficulties in his reference point to the outside world. A patient with this difficulty may have trouble using his contralateral limbs, may confuse the sides of the body, and may not differentiate properly his own body parts and those of the examiner.[4,7,8,10]

Macro- and microsomatognosia are disorders in body scheme that distort a person's perception of his own body. A patient may see his whole body or part of it as abnormally small (micro) or exceptionally large (macro).

In patients who have somatognosia without an accompanying problem in spatial relations, the prospects for successfully attaining skills of daily living are high.

Evaluation of Somatognosia

TEST 1: POINT TO BODY PARTS ON COMMAND[11-14]

Description:
Therapist asks patient to point or indicate in some way the body part named on himself, on the examiner, and on a human figure, puzzle, or doll. There is no standardized form for this test. The therapist can make up the commands. Here are some examples excluding "left" and "right" from the command.
1. Show me your knees.
2. Show me your mouth.
3. Show me your stomach.
4. Show me your nose.
5. Show me your feet.
6. Show me your shoulders.
7. Show me your elbows.
8. Show me your hair.
9. Show me your back.

Scoring:
Nonstandardized.
Intact — patient correctly indicates all parts named in a reasonable length of time.

Validity:
Sauguet, Macdonald and Boone[11,13,15,16] use variations of this to measure body scheme. It is used mainly to test a patient's verbal understanding. Sauguet separated his sample into left hemiplegics, right hemiplegics without receptive aphasia, and right hemiplegics with

receptive aphasia. Only the patients with receptive aphasia made errors on this test. Boone found that if the words "right" and "left" were excluded from the command, most of the errors were eliminated.

Reliability:
Research conducted with adult patients sustaining head trauma on a variation of this test established inter-rater reliability (r=0.94).[17] Item analysis of this subtest given with four additional subtests (ie, Draw-A-Person, Right/Left Discrimination, Body Puzzle and Face Puzzle) indicated good internal consistency (coefficient alpha = 0.60).[17*]
To improve validity, rule out aphasia as a cause of poor performance.

TEST 2: POINT TO BODY PARTS—IMITATION[1,16]

Description:
The patient is told to imitate movements of the examiner, who touches different parts of his own body. Mirror image responses are acceptable. There is no standardized form of this test. Therapists can make up their own commands. Touching six to ten body parts is sufficient. For example:
1. Touch your left hand.
2. Touch your right cheek.
3. Touch your left leg.
4. Touch your left elbow.
5. Touch your right palm.
6. Touch your right knee.
7. Touch your left shoulder.
8. Touch your right ear.
9. Touch your right forearm.
10. Touch your left wrist.

Scoring:
Nonstandardized.
Intact—patient correctly indicates all parts named within a reasonable length of time.

Validity:
This test eliminates most of the verbal problems of the last test. Indeed, in Sauguet's[16] study, 90 percent of the right hemiplegics with aphasia had a normal performance, as compared with 100 percent of the right hemiplegics without aphasia and left hemiplegics.
To improve validity, rule out apraxia as a cause of poor performance.

TEST 3A: BODY VISUALIZATION AND SPACE CONCEPTS

(Norm descriptive statistics available in adaptation by Taylor)[18†]

Description:
The examiner reads questions to the patient. Instruct the patient to "Think of yourself sitting as you are now when answering the following questions."
1. Ordinarily, are a person's teeth inside or outside his mouth?
2. Are your legs below your stomach?
3. Which is farther from your nose—your feet or your stomach?
4. Is your mouth above your eyes?
5. Which is closer to your mouth—your neck or shoulder?

---

*A coefficient alpha measure of 0.50 was considered acceptable for the establishment of reliability.

---

†Developed by A.M. Ayres, ADI Auxiliary Publication Project, Document 8179, Library of Congress, Washington, DC.

6. Is your shoulder between your neck and your elbow?
7. Are your fingers between your elbow and your hand?
8. Which is farther from your toes—your heel or elbow?
9. Which is nearer to your head—your arms or your legs?
10. Which is on top of your head—your hair or eyes?
11. Is your back behind you or in front of you?
12. Is your stomach behind you or in front of you?
13. Is your elbow above or below your shoulder?
14. Is your nose above or below your neck?

Scoring:
Although this test has not been standardized for adults, Taylor[19] provides the data in Table 5-1. However, until a more extensive normative study can be done, interpretation of scores is nonstandardized.

Intact — patient correctly answers all questions within a reasonable length of time. To improve validity, rule out aphasia as a cause of poor performance.

TABLE 5-1

Age	Number of Subjects	Mean Score	Standard Division
50-64	90	27.5	1.3
65-74	60	26.9	1.2

TEST 3B: BODY REVISUALIZATION
Macdonald[13] has devised a shorter version of this test in which the patient only has to answer "true" or "false." An expressive aphasia patient can indicate "true" or "false" by pointing to one of two cards marked "true" and "false."

Description:
Ask the patient whether these statements are true or false:
1. Your mouth is below your chin.
2. Your eyes are above your forehead.
3. Your knees are below your hips.
4. Your hands are at the end of your arms.
5. You have one chin, one nose, and one mouth.

Scoring:
Nonstandardized.
Intact—all correct within a reasonable length of time. To improve validity, rule out receptive aphasia.

TEST 4: DRAW-A-MAN[13,20,21]

Description:
Patient is given a blank piece of paper and a pencil and is asked to draw a man.

Scoring:
Nonstandardized.
The following scoring system is taken from Macdonald.[13] The Goodenough-Harris Drawing Test[22] and the Denver Developmental Screening Test[23] both have standardized scoring systems for children. The first is more complicated than Macdonald's; the second is less complicated. The second scoring system included in this section is from Zoltan et al.[14]

Scoring System No. 1:
1. Total of four points for presence of all body parts.
   Point distribution:
   > a. One point—head
   > b. One point—trunk
   > c. Two points—two arms if full figure, one arm if profile
   > d. Two points—two legs if full figure, one leg if profile
2. Total of three points for correct proportion of body parts to trunk.
   Point distribution:
   > a. One point — area of head not more than one-half or less than one-half the length of the trunk
   > b. One point — at least one arm not longer than twice the length of the trunk or less than one-half the length of the trunk
   > c. One point — at least one leg not longer than twice the length of the trunk or less than the length of the trunk.
3. Total of one point for correct postural alignment, ie, figure in normal standing or sitting position.
4. Total of two points for correct juxtaposition of extremities with trunk.
   Point distribution:
   > a. One point—arms emerge from upper one-half of trunk
   > b. One point—legs emerge from lower one-half of trunk
   > Intact—total score of 10 points

Scoring System No. 2:
Total of 10 body parts:

Head	Right hand
Trunk	Left hand
Right arm	Right foot
Left arm	Left foot
Right leg	Left leg

Intact—scores 10
Minimally impaired—scores 6 to 9
Severely impaired—scores 5 or below

Reliability:
Research conducted on a sample of patients with head trauma utilizing this scoring system established inter-rater reliability (r=0.86).[17] As noted with the pointing to body parts test, the Draw-A-Person Test, when given to adult patients with head trauma with four other sub-tests, had an overall reliability of coefficient alpha = 0.60.[17]

To improve validity:
This test is also used as a means of identifying or diagnosing unilateral neglect and anosognosia. It is a constructional task and therefore overlaps into disorders of spatial judgment and apraxia, which should be ruled out. The validity of this test as a test of body scheme is controversial. Maloney and Payne[21] treated a group of developmentally delayed teenagers with sensory-motor training based on the work of Kephart, and pre- and post-tested them with three tests of body image including the Draw-A-Man Test. On the post-testing, the group made significant gains on the two other tests of body image but not on the Draw-A-Man Test. They concluded that the test does not reflect changes in body image occurring as a result of sensory-motor training. The Draw-A-Man Test is also used as a personality projective test, ie, to determine how one feels about one's body. Gregory and Aitken[20] found that depressed patients often drew a miserable looking man whose size was very small on the page. This test is also used as a test of intelligence.[22]

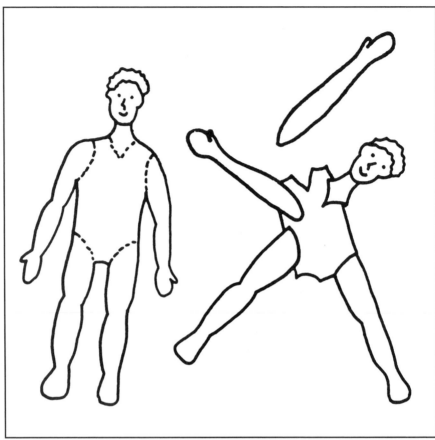

Figure 5-1. Left, human figure puzzle. Right, example of a severely impaired performance.

TEST 5: HUMAN FIGURE OR FACE PUZZLE[13,14,20]
(Figure 5-1)

Equipment:
- Pieces of felt or cardboard or Plexiglas cut out to represent head, trunk, arms, legs, hands and feet
- Large piece of black felt for background

Description:
The patient is asked to put together pieces to resemble a human figure after individual parts have first been identified for the patient. For example, "Here are the man's arms, legs, head, and trunk. See whether you can put him together." In a variation of this test, the patient is not told that it is a man, but simply told to put the puzzle together.

Scoring:
Subjective, nonstandardized.[14]
Intact—able to assemble puzzle in 1.5 minutes with no errors
Impaired—able to put four to ten pieces together but takes more than 1.5 minutes
Severely impaired—able to put one to three pieces together correctly

Reliability:
Research conducted on a sample of patients with head trauma utilizing this scoring system

established inter-rater reliability (r=0.84).[17] As noted with the previous body scheme tests, when given with the four other subtests, the overall reliability was good (alpha = 0.60).[17] To improve validity, rule out spatial-constructional disorders and figure-ground problems as causes of poor performance. This test is also used to test unilateral neglect and anosognosia.

TEST 6: FACE PUZZLE[24]

Description:
The patient is asked to put together pieces to resemble a human face.

Scoring:
Nonstandardized.
To improve validity, rule out constructional disorders and figure-ground problems as causes of poor performance.

Reliability:
Research conducted on a sample of patients with head trauma indicated no variation in subject performance and a high correlation with constructional praxis.[17]
Future research should indicate whether this is a meaningful test of body scheme.

Treatment for Somatognosia

Utilizing a Remedial Approach:

1. Provide tactile input/stimulation, eg, have the patient rub his arm with a rough cloth while naming the body part.
2. Practice particular tasks that reinforce body knowledge. For example:
    a. The patient identifies body parts as they are touched by the therapist.
    b. Quiz the patient on body parts; eg, "Show me or touch your knees."
    c. Patient practices putting together a human figure.
3. Apply concepts from the neurodevelopmental frame of reference as follows:
    a. Incorporate into treatment bilateral activities that facilitate normal movement, forced use of the affected extremity, and improved body scheme.
    b. Provide appropriate handling techniques to educate the patient about what it feels like to move normally. Provide treatment in a variety of ways and positions to facilitate retention of motor learning.

Utilizing an Adaptive Approach:

1. Identify where in the body knowledge representation the breakdown occurs. Educate the patient and his family regarding the patient's body scheme deficits and how they affect function. Train the family in how to assist the patient in affected self-care tasks in order to compensate.
2. If the patient has a functional awareness of body parts but not a spatial awareness, or vice versa, utilize this in your approach and patient cuing to maximize function. For example: "Move the part of the body that you use to hold things," instead of "Move your hand."

3. If the patient is able to localize a body part near the correct one (ie, pointing to shoulder when asked to point to arm), utilize this in your approach and patient cuing. For example, if you ask the patient to move his arm and he moves his shoulder, say, "Move the part of your body just below the one you just moved."

Unilateral Body Neglect

Unilateral body neglect is the inability to integrate and use perceptions from one (usually left) side of the body.[25] This deficit may occur independently of visual field cuts or visual inattention or be compounded by these deficits. The patient with unilateral body neglect will ignore one half of his body. For example, a male subject may forget to shave one side of his face or forget to dress one side of his body.

Evaluation for Unilateral Body Neglect

TEST 1: DRAW-A-MAN

Description:
Patient is given separate sheets of blank paper for each task and told to draw a man.

Scoring:
Subjective.
Intact—drawings include all parts in proper place.
Impaired—some parts are missing from the left side, or body parts are thinner on left side, or parts are skewed to the right.
To improve validity, rule out constructional and motor apraxias.

TEST 2: FUNCTIONAL

Description:
Probably the best test of unilateral body neglect is observation during functional activities. Does the patient ignore one half of his body while performing self-care activities such as brushing teeth, shaving or dressing?

Scoring:
Subjective.
Intact—patient shows no signs of unilateral body neglect during self-care activities.
Impaired—patient shows signs of unilateral body neglect in some, but not all self-care activities.
Severely Impaired—patient shows signs of unilateral body neglect in all self-care activities.

Treatment for Unilateral Body Neglect
Utilizing a Remedial Approach:

1. Provide tactile or proprioceptive stimulation to the neglected side prior to self-care tasks. For example:
    a. Therapist rubs affected arm of patient while patient watches, using either his own hand, a rough cloth, or vibrator.

b. Patient rubs himself with his nonaffected hand while he watches it.

c. While watching himself, patient self-ranges the affected arm and hand to assist if he has little muscle power.

2. Apply concepts from a neurodevelopmental frame of reference. Have the patient participate in bilateral tasks to facilitate increased total body awareness. Specific handling techniques and proprioceptive facilitation through weight bearing activities will also help. Set up activities which will "force the use" of the neglected extremities.

3. Apply concepts from an Affolter frame of reference. Provide tactile kinesthetic guiding during self-care tasks.

Utilizing an Adaptive Approach:

1. Educate the patient and his family about the patient's unilateral body neglect and how it will affect function. Train the family in how to assist the patient in affected self-care tasks in order to compensate. Highlight activities where safety is an issue.

2. Provide visual cues or reminders to the patient. For example, a sign on the patient's mirror reading, "Have I shaved both sides of my face?" or "Have I washed both arms?"

3. Provide verbal cuing to the patient during self-care tasks as needed to compensate for body neglect.

4. Train the patient to self-monitor his performance. For example, after he feels he has completed a task such as putting on a shirt, he asks himself, "Have I put each arm through a sleeve?" or after shaving the patient asks, "Have I shaved both sides of my face?" The patient should then check himself if he has completed the task correctly before moving on to the next task. If necessary, the patient could utilize a daily activity checklist to monitor his performance after task completion.

Anosognosia

Anosognosia is a relatively transient, severe form of neglect to the extent that the patient fails to recognize the presence of severity of his paralysis.[26,27] Anosognosia may be simply unconcern for the paralysis (anosodiaphoria) or, at the other extreme, may be a complete denial of paralysis. When asked whether anything is wrong, the patient denies his illness.[28] If confronted by the fact that the side is paralyzed and will not move in response to his efforts, the patient may reply that the limb has "a will and purpose of its own,"[20] that "it is tired," or that "it always was a lazy arm."

The patient with anosognosia is unable to form a consistent and accurate picture of the reality of his paralysis.[29] The deficit is often associated with mental confusion or intellectual impairments; however, the deficit may occur independently.[26] The lack of awareness may be evident in the patient's verbal or nonverbal behavior. Many anosognostic patients also have visual neglect.[29] Denial may take the form of confabulation, and the patient will persist in his belief despite repeated demonstration of disability.[27] As the denial decreases, the patient may become agitated, frustrated and/or depressed.

It has been recently theorized that anosognosia requires both cognitive impairment and sensory, especially proprioceptive loss.[29] The awareness of a sensorimotor deficit is hypothesized not as an immediate sensory phenomenon, but rather as a result of discovery or the product of observation and inference. The anosognostic patient cannot make any inference of why he cannot perform a task. His reasoning skills are impaired. Levine hypothesizes "that cognitive deficits impairing the ability to infer will distinguish those individuals with sensory loss and paralysis who are anosognosic from those who discover and become aware of their paralysis."[29]

Montague Ullman[30] has attempted to interpret anosognosia as a way in which the patient experiences his body. Even transient C.V.A. patients have described a limb as feeling like it is "not there" or not belonging to the body. In a patient with brain damage, abstract thinking may be diminished so that he is tied to subjective experience. Thus, if the arm does not feel a part of him or does not hurt, he cannot make reasonable judgments about it. Another variable is the patient's premorbid personality; that is, the patient may have always been one to go through life verbally denying that anything was wrong no matter what the crisis or disturbing event. With these two factors working together, the patient does not have to deal with an illness he cannot perceive, and also can separate himself from a stressful situation. In his way, the patient is preserving his own intactness. The following example illustrates these concepts:[30]

A patient lying in bed noticed his arm protruding from a blanket. He remarked spontaneously, "When I was put in bed, this arm was sticking out. I told the nurses and doctors. They think it's my arm, but it's not. That's been sticking out like this ever since I was put in here."

"Whose hand is it?"

"I wouldn't know. It was here when they put me in bed. I always had an idea I was laying on top of a corpse because this hand was lying out there motionless."

Evaluation for Anosognosia

There are no standardized assessments specific to anosognosia. Please refer to the evaluation section in Chapter 9 on decreased awareness for assessments, which includes a portion devoted to decreased sensory motor awareness. Generally, the therapist should record relevant spontaneous behavior as well as behavior as a result of his inquiries.[26]

Treatment for Anosognosia

Please refer to treatment suggestions in Chapter 9 for decreased awareness.

Right-Left Discrimination

Right-left discrimination is a skill that develops relatively late.[6] In most people, it is not mastered until seven years of age or later.[31] The patient who has sustained a C.V.A. or T.B.I. may exhibit difficulty with right-left discrimination. This difficulty is generally characterized by a selective incapacity to apply the right-left distinction to symmetrical parts of the body.[32] It is a specific disorder of spatial orientation "restricted to the sagittal plane of the subject's body or that of the confronting examiner."[32]

Generally associated with parietal lobe dysfunction, right-left disorientation is considered by some to be a rare but striking disorder.[6] It is generally evaluated by assessing the patient's ability to point to the side of the body indicated by the therapist on verbal command or imitation.[5] The skills required for this assessment are verbal, sensory and conceptual.[32] The patient must understand the term and retain it in short-term memory for the time necessary to execute the command. The patient must also be able to discriminate sensory input from the opposite one. Finally, for tasks which involve right-left discrimination on others, the patient must be able to manipulate his personal orientation, which requires a high degree of conceptual skill.

Evaluation of Right-Left Discrimination

TEST 1: AYRES' RIGHT-LEFT DISCRIMINATION TEST
(subtest of the Southern California Sensory Integration Tests)[33]

Description:
Therapist sits facing the patient and gives the patient a series of commands.
1. Show me your right hand.
2. Touch your left ear.
3. Take this pencil with your right hand. (Hold pencil in both hands, hands resting on knees.)
4. Now put it in my right hand. (Holds hands palm up on knees.)
5. Is this pencil on your right or left side? (Hold pencil in left hand one foot in front of patient's right shoulder.)
6. Touch your right eye.
7. Show me your left foot.
8. Is this pencil on your right or left side? (Hold pencil in right hand in front of patient's left shoulder.)
9. Take this pencil with your left hand. (Hold pencil in both hands, hands resting on knees.)
10. Now, put it in my left hand. (Hold hands palm up on knees.)

Scoring:
Score two points if correct within 3 seconds and one point if correct within 4 to 10 seconds. If patient first makes a wrong response and then corrects himself, the score is based on the time of correct response. If the command is repeated, the score can be no more than one. This test has been standardized only for children. In testing its reliability for children aged 4.0 to 8.11 years, the test-retest correlations ranged from r=0.15 to 0.54. Scoring for adults is nonstandardized.
Intact—as adult norms have not been established, the therapist should gather his or her own provisional norms by testing a few normal adults.
To improve validity, rule out aphasia and apraxia.

Reliability:
Inter-rater reliability (r=0.93) was established for this test on a sample of adult head trauma patients.[17]

TEST 2: POINT TO BODY PARTS ON COMMAND[16]

Description:
The therapist asks the patient to point or indicate in some way the body parts named on himself, on the examiner, or on a human figure doll or puzzle. There is no standardized form of this test. The therapist can make up his or her own. For example:
1. Show me your left hand.
2. Show me your right eye.

3.   Show me your left foot.
4.   Show me your left shoulder.
5.   Show me your right elbow.
6.   Show me your left knee.
7.   Show me your right ear.
8.   Show me your left wrist.
9.   Show me your right ankle.
10.   Show me your right thumb.

Scoring:
Nonstandardized.
Intact—patient correctly indicates all parts named within a reasonable length of time.
To improve validity, rule out aphasia and apraxia as causes of poor performance. This is similar to Test 1 under Somatognosia, except that the words "left" and "right" are included in the commands. The two tests could be combined by using commands with and without "left" and "right" in them. One could then compare the results. Does the patient do better with commands omitting "left" and "right"? Does he indicate the correct body part but on the wrong side, ie, lift left hand when commanded to "Show me your right hand"? Then it is a problem of right-left discrimination. If the patient is totally confused and indicates the wrong body part altogether, it may be a problem of somatognosia.

Reliability:
Inter-rater reliability (r=0.94) was established for a variation of this test on a sample of adult patients with head trauma.[17]

Treatment for Right-Left Discrimination

Utilizing a Remedial Approach:

1.   Provide extra tactile and proprioceptive input during activities. For example, a weighted cuff on the dominant wrist.

Utilizing an Adaptive Approach:

1.   Identify what areas of occupational performance are impacted by the patient's difficulty with right-left discrimination. Provide adaptations for these activities to help the patient compensate. For example, wearing a watch on a certain wrist consistently, a marking on clothing, shoes or other necessary items with colored tape or marker to distinguish right from left.
2.   When giving instructions to the patient, do not use the words "right" or "left." Either point or refer to the item by its location. For example, "Your comb is next to your toothbrush."

Finger Agnosia

Finger agnosia consists of doubt and hesitation concerning the fingers. A fairly common occurrence, it is usually found bilaterally, with more involvement of the three middle fingers of each hand. The patient has confusion in naming his fingers on command or knowing which one was touched.[20,34] Patients with finger agnosia will often display clumsiness in using fin-

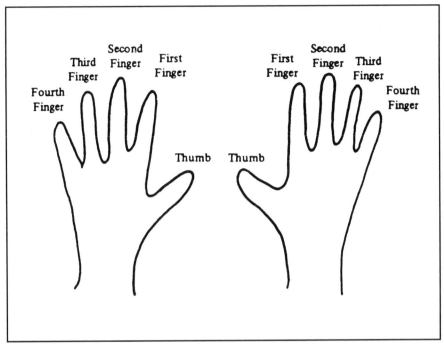

Figure 5-2. Hand chart for Tests 1 and 2 under Figure Agnosia (reduced from life size).

gers, especially in tasks requiring imitation of meaningful gestures.[35] Deficits in finger agnosia have been found to correlate highly with poor dexterity in tasks involving movement of the fingers in relation to each other. Some theorists have questioned why the fingers have assumed an unusual significance in body scheme disorders.[6] Some theorize it is because the fingers are the principle means of touch. Others believe it is because of its importance in reaching and as a marker for fine spatial coordinates.[6] Still others focus on the key role of the hand as an executive tool for visuomotor coordination.

Finger agnosia has traditionally been linked with Gerstmann's syndrome.[1,34] This syndrome includes finger agnosia, impaired right-left discrimination, agraphia and acalculia. Recent documentation however, has described the component parts of the syndrome as seen independently.[1] It is assumed by others that finger agnosia is not a primary deficit, but part of an associated intellectual impairment and aphasia.[1] Finally, some theorize that finger agnosia is a disorder of spatial orientation, with respect to the actual sequence of the fingers of the hand.[34]

Evaluation for Finger Agnosia

TEST 1: FINGER LOCALIZATION — NAMING[13,16]

Description:
Have the patient place his hands palm down on the table. A picture of two hands (Figure 5-2) is placed in front of the patient so that the fingers in the picture point in the same direction as the patient's fingers. The therapist touches the patient's fingers one at a time, saying, "I am going to touch your fingers one at a time. Name or point to the finger on the picture of the hand that is the same as the finger I touched."

This test can be given with the patient watching while he is touched and with vision occluded. A combination of both—five items with vision and five with vision occluded—is useful to compare results. To occlude vision, the therapist can ask the patient to close his eyes, or shield his eyes with a file folder, or ask the patient to place his hands in a specially made box that has two ends open, one end covered with a curtain so that the patient cannot see in. There is no standardized form of this test. The therapist can make up his or her own order. For example: "Which finger am I touching?" Touch the patient with a pencil eraser on his:

1. Right second finger
2. Left third finger.
3. Right thumb.
4. Left fourth finger.
5. Right first finger.
6. Left second finger.
7. Right fourth finger.
8. Left first finger
9. Right third finger.
10. Left first finger.

Scoring:
Nonstandardized.
Intact—patient correctly indicates all fingers touched within a reasonable length of time.
To improve validity, rule out impaired sensation on both hands.

TEST 2: FINGER IDENTIFICATION BY NAME[13,16]

Description:
The patient is asked to move or point to the finger on his own hand named by the therapist. A variation of this test is to have the patient point to the finger on his hand matching the one the therapist points to on the hand chart (see Figure 5-2). This test is not standardized. The therapist can make up his or her own order. Five to 10 commands is probably sufficient. For an example, see Test 1 under Finger Agnosia.

Scoring:
Nonstandardized.
Intact—patient correctly indicates all fingers named within a reasonable length of time.
To improve validity, rule out aphasia.

TEST 3: IMITATION[16]

Description:
Patient is instructed to imitate finger movements made by the therapist. There is no standardized form of this test. The therapist can make up her own movements. Five movements are sufficient. For example:

1. Therapist curls right index finger forward.
2. Therapist touches left thumb to tip of left little finger.
3. Therapist touches left middle finger with tip of right index finger.
4. Therapist brings left index and middle fingers together laterally.
5. Therapist circumducts right thumb.

Scoring:
Subjective.
Intact—patient imitates all movements correctly within a reasonable length of time. To improve validity, rule out apraxia, abnormal muscle tone and paralysis/paresis of affected hand.

Treatment for Finger Agnosia

Utilizing a Remedial Approach:

Apply the following concepts and techniques:[36]

1. Representation of the body in the cortex is use dependent, therefore treatment should be structured so that repeated sensory inputs are provided to those surfaces to be used for the desired task, ie, fingertips and thumbpad.

2. Repeated sensory stimulation should be high intensity for appreciation but not aversive. For example, a thin band of Velcro is stroked across the key sensory surfaces first with patient's eyes open, then closed. The patient is asked to identify which finger is being stimulated.

3. Subsequent to the stimulation, have the patient perform a functional hand or ADL activity appropriate to his level of function, ie, holding an adapted fork, dressing, etc.

4. The first skills needed are to grip an object with the appropriate amount of pressure while holding, depending on the object. If the patient's finger agnosia has affected this skill, provide small lateral movements of the skin against an object (shear or friction). This type of stimulation has been found to be more effective in activating deep structures or muscle input than direct vertical pressure.[36]

Cortical reorganization is enhanced when the patient is motivated and attentive. Make the stimulus relevant to the patient's daily life. For example, if the patient is an avid golfer, use grasp of a golf club or manipulation of a golf ball.

Utilizing an Adaptive Approach:

1. Educate the patient and his family as to how the finger agnosia may affect dexterity and function. Highlight areas where safety is an issue. Provide environmental adaptations as needed. For example, adaptive handles or Velcro covered keys on a computer keyboard.

References

1. Cumming WJK. The neurobiology of the body schema. *British Journal of Psychiatry.* 1988;153(2):7-11.

2. Reed CL, Farah MJ. The psychological reality of the body schema: A test with normal participants. *J Exp Psych Hum Perc Perf.* 1995;21(2): 334-343.

3. Semenza C, Goodglass H. Localization of body parts in brain injured subjects. *Neuropsychologia.* 1985;23(2):161-175.

4. Zoltan B. Visual, visual perceptual and perceptual-motor deficits in brain injured adults: Evaluation, treatment and functional implications. In: Kraft GH, Berrol S. (eds). *Physical Medicine and Rehabilitation Clinics of North America.* Philadelphia, WB Saunders Co.; 1992.

5. Van Deusen J. Unilateral neglect: Suggestions for research by occupational therapists. *Amer J Occup Ther.* 1988;42(7):441-446.

6. Newcombe F, Ratcliff G. Disorders of visuospatial analysis. In: Boller F, Grafman J (eds). *Handbook of Neuropsychology* (Vol. 2). Amsterdam, Elsevier Science Pubs.; 1989.

7. Zoltan B. Remediation of visual-perceptual and perceptual-motor deficits. In: Rosenthal M, Griffith ER, Bond MR, Miller JD (eds.). *Rehabilitation of the Adult and Child with Traumatic Brain Injury.* Philadelphia, FA Davis Co.; 1990.

8. Sirigu A, Grafman J, Bressler K, Sunderland T. Multiple representations contribute to body knowledge processing: Evidence from a case of autotopagnosia. *Brain.* 1991;114:629-642.

9. Hansen CS. Traumatic brain injury. In: Van Deusen J. (ed). *Body Image and Perceptual Dysfunction in Adults.* Philadelphia, WB Saunders; 1993.

10. Parker RS. *Traumatic Brain Injury and Neuropsychological Impairment.* New York, Springer-Verlag; 1990.

11. Boone D, Landes B. Left-right discrimination in hemiplegic patients. *Arch Phys Med.* 1968;49:533-537.

12. Brown AL. Motivation to learn and understand: On taking charge of one's own learning. *Cognition and Instruction.* 1988;5:311-321.

13. Macdonald J. An investigation of body scheme in adults with cerebral vascular accident. *Am J Occup Ther.* 1960;14:72-79.

14. Zoltan B, Jabri J, Panikoff L, Ryckman D. *Perceptual Motor Evaluation for Head Injured and Other Neurologically Impaired Adults.* San Jose, California. Santa Clara Valley Medical Center, Occupational Therapy Department; 1983.

15. Brown J. *Aphasia, Apraxia and Agnosia: Clinical and Theoretical Aspects.* Springfield, Illinois, Charles C. Thomas Pub.; 1972.

16. Sauguet J, Benton AL, Hecaen H. Disturbances of the body scheme in relation to language impairment and hemispheric locus of lesion. *J Neurol Neurosurg Psychiat.* 1971;34:496-501.

17. Baum B. The establishment of reliability and validity of a perceptual evaluation on a sample of adult head trauma patients. Thesis, University of Southern California, December 1981.

18. Taylor MM. Controlled evaluation of percept-concept—motor training therapy after stroke resulting in left hemiplegia. Research grant RD-2215-M, sponsored by Rehabilitation Institute, Detroit, September 1969.

19. Taylor MM. Analysis of dysfunction in the left hemiplegia following stroke. *Am J Occup Ther.* 1968;22:512-520.

20. Gregory ME, Aitkin JA. Assessment of parietal lobe function in hemiplegia. *Occup Ther.* 1971;34:9-17.

21. Maloney MP, Payne L. Validity of the draw-a-person test as a measure of body image. *Percept Motor Skills.* 1969;29:119-122.

22. Goodenough F, Harris D. *Goodenough-Harris Drawing Test.* New York, Harcourt, Brace & World; 1963.

23. Frankenberg WK, Dods JB. *Denver Developmental Screening Test.* Denver, Ladoca Project and Publishing Foundation, Inc.; 1970.

24. Wall N, et al. *Hemiplegic Evaluation.* Boston, Massachusetts Rehabilitation Hospital; 1979.

25. Bouska MJ, Kauffman NA, Marcus, SE. Disorders of the visual perceptual system. In: Umphred DA (ed). *Neurological Rehabilitation (2nd edition).* St. Louis, CV Mosby Co.; 1990.

26. Bisiach E, Geminiani G. Anosognosia related to hemiplegia and hemianopia. In: Prigatano GP, Schacter DL (eds.). *Awareness of Defects After Brain Injury.* New York, Oxford University Press; 1991.

27. Weinstein EA. Anosognosia and denial of illness. In: Prigitano GP, Schacter DL (eds.). *Awareness of Deficits After Injury.* New York, Oxford University Press; 1991.

28. Sawtell R, Martin G. Perceptual problems of the hemiplegic patient. *Lancet.* 1967;87:193-196.

29. Levine DA. Unawareness of visual and sensorimotor defects: A hypothesis. *Brain and Cognition.* 1990;13:233-281.

30. Ullman M. Disorder of body image after stroke. *Am J Nurs.* 1964;64:89-91.

31. Kosslyn SM, Koenig O, Barrett A, Backer-Cave C, Tang J, Gabrieli JDE. Evidence for two types of spatial representations: Hemispheric specialization for categorical and coordinate relations. *J Exp Psych: Hum Percept Perform.* 1989;15(4):723-735.

32. Benton A. *Right-Left Discrimination and Finger Localization.* New York, Harper Bros.; 1959.

33. Ayres AJ. *Southern California Sensory Integration Tests.* Los Angeles, Western Psychological Services; 1972.

34. Benton AL. Gerstmann's syndrome. *Arch Neurol.* 1992;49:445-447.

35. Benson DF. Disorders of Visual Gnosis. In: Brown JW (ed.). *Neuropsychology of Visual Perception.* New Jersey, Lawrence Erllaum Assoc.; 1989.

36. Dannenbaum RM, Jones LA. The assessment and treatment of patients who have sensory loss following cortical lesions. *J Hand Therapy*. April-June 1993:130-138.

CHAPTER 6

Visual Discrimination Skills

Form Discrimination

The ability to distinguish different types of forms is an important ability for successful environmental interaction. It plays an important role in visual recognition of objects, in visually guided manipulations, and in navigation within the environment.[1] The perception of spatial properties such as form is accomplished immediately and effortlessly. Color, orientation, edge and motion cues are all utilized for form discrimination.[2-5] Difficulties with form perception have been associated with parietal and temporal lobe damage.[2,6]

Many theorists believe that form perception is accomplished by two processes with two separate systems, carrying different aspects of form information.[2-4] The first system is hypothesized to perform abstract processing to recognize types of forms. The second system provides specific processing to distinguish different instances of a type of form. These two systems operate relatively independently within the brain.[4]

The Abstract Visual Form system (AVF) is utilized when visual form information should be processed and stored in an abstract, nonspecific manner.[4] For example, when an individual is scanning a cluttered desk to find a writing instrument to write a phone message, he is attempting to identify a pencil, but not necessarily a particular pencil. This is accomplished by the AVF system, which distinguishes between different types of forms.

The Specific Visual Form system (SVF), on the other hand, produces specific output representations. It processes input in a manner that preserves visual details to produce output representations that distinguish different instances of the same type of form. For instance, identifying a particular, familiar pencil with which to write.

It is further hypothesized that the visual form systems process visual structure information during perception and subsequently store it in long-term "modality specific" information centers about visual form. The conceptual information associated with this structural information is not stored with it.[4] This concept of a specific center or centers that are the "form areas" exclusively has recently been challenged. Research has indicated there are a large number of cortical regions which are active during different form tasks.[2]

A disorder in form perception involves an inability to attend to subtle variations in form. The patient may mistake a water pitcher for a urinal or a button for a nickel.

Evaluation for Form Discrimination

TEST 1: FORMBOARD TEST[7]

Procedure:
Show the patient the ten forms and test plate. Hand the patient one form at a time, telling him to match each shape on the boards. The therapist may give a demonstration for aphasic patients. Take the form out of eyesight after the patient has matched it, so that he cannot use the process of elimination.

Directions:
"Place each form on the shape that matches it."
Observe for spatial neglect, perseveration, poor planning or comprehension, and general inability to deal with objects.

Score:
Severely impaired — unable to match more than one to four forms.
Impaired — able to match five to nine forms.
Intact — matches all ten forms correctly.
To improve validity, rule out poor vision, visual field loss, poor color discrimination, and constructional apraxia as causes of poor performance.

Reliability:
Inter-rater reliability (r=1.0) was established for this test on a sample of adult patients with head trauma.[8]

TEST 2: FUNCTIONAL

Description:
Observe the patient during various activities and note whether he has difficulty distinguishing between different objects of similar forms, ie, eating utensils in the kitchen.

Scoring:
Subjective. The instances when and where difficulty was observed are recorded.
Intact — patient displays no difficulty in distinguishing forms during occupational performance tasks.

Treatment for Form Discrimination

Utilizing a Remedial Approach:

1. Have the patient match similar parquetry block forms.
2. Have the patient practice sorting functional objects such as kitchen utensils.
3. For activities such as #1 or #2, have the patient use tactile cues by feeling objects for successful task completion.
4. Place Velcro strips on elevated surfaces of specific objects with distinct edges.[9] Train the patient to explore with the fingers both the location and form of the objects covered with Velcro. The patient should perform the task first with his eyes open, then closed.

5. Inputs should be applied to have enhanced contrast, ie, feeling a moving or irregular input passed through the hand.[9]

Utilizing an Adaptive Approach:

1. Shapes are best recognized with an upright orientation; therefore, place items necessary to the patient's function in the upright position.[5,10] For example, hang garden tools up separately instead of piled in a drawer
2. Label important items that the patient is unable to distinguish.
3. Organize items and maintain this organization so the patient can distinguish items by location.

Depth Perception (Stereopsis)

Depth perception, or stereopsis, is crucial to the individual's ability to locate objects in the visual environment, to have accurate hand movements under visual guidance, and to function safely with tasks such as navigating stairs or driving.[11,12] Stereopsis has been defined as the "ability to visualize the third dimension of depth."[13] Human stereopsis is evident at about two months of age. The process of stereopsis, generally associated with right hemisphere dominance,[14] is considered relatively low level because "the neural mechanisms for the binocular extraction of depth occur early in the cortical hierarchy of visuospatial functions."[11] Stereopsis does not appear to depend on visual recognition and does not need to be taught. However, depth is a perceptual attribute and therefore cannot be arrived at without the participation of the observer.[15]

The theoretical basis of depth perception acquisition has emphasized areas such as the fusion of information from two monocular views, and binocular rivalry or suppression.[11,13,16] The perception of depth has also recently been linked to the sensitivity of the visual system to spatial frequency information.[17] Classic stereopsis relies on the fact that "two physical points in space lying at different distances lead to differential retinal disparity of the two pairs of binocular image points."[16] Binocular disparity is the most important cue for depth perception.[18] More specifically, horizontal disparity is the crucial input for stereopsis. Vertical disparity does not contribute to stereopsis "although large vertical disparities must be corrected prior to stereopsis by vertical vergence eye movements."[11]

Horizontal spatial disparity is only one disparity cue for stereopsis. Temporal disparity and intraocular differences in brightness may also contribute.[11] In addition, recent research has focused on the formation of subjective occluding contours and surface resulting from unpaired points in binocular images. As Nakayama & Shimojo[16] describe, "distant surfaces are occluded by nearer surfaces to different extents in the two eyes, leading to the existence of unpaired image points visible in one eye and not the other." These researchers believe the visual system utilizes the occlusive relations in the real world to recover depth, contour and surface from unpaired points.

The concept of binocular rivalry or suppression has also been explored. Some theorize that "when stimuli are rivalrous, one or the other may predominate in alternating fashion."[11] The "losing" image is thought to be suppressed. Due to this binocular suppression, the individual is unaware of the discordant view of the two eyes in normal viewing when fixating on a near object. Depth information related to objects in the visual environment are derived from monocular cues such as "linear perspective, texture, gradients and apparent size of familiar objects."[11] For example, when an object is farther away in depth, it will appear smaller. In addition, less detail will be evident than when it is closer in depth.[17]

As a result of T.B.I., it is common for the patient to have fusion and no diplopia (double vision) and yet have no depth perception.[13] Stereopsis may be impaired without strabismus as a result of damage in the visual cortices through a C.V.A. or T.B.I.[11]

The evaluation of depth perception has traditionally included asking the patient to estimate distance in the natural environment, to judge the relative distance of real three dimensional objects under more controlled conditions, and by measuring the acuity of stereoscopic vision.[14] Examples of these evaluation methods are described below.

Evaluation of Depth Perception

TEST 1: BLOCKS

Description:
The therapist lines up a row of small cube blocks so that they are perpendicular to the patient. The patient is asked in turn, "Which block is nearest?" "Which block is farthest away?" and "Which block is in the middle?" The questions are repeated after the therapist has moved the blocks so that they are lined up diagonally to the patient.

Scoring:
Subjective.
Intact —patient correctly identifies each block asked for.
To improve validity, rule out aphasia. Make sure the patient understands the concepts "nearest," "farthest away," and "in the middle."

Reliability:
In a study of adult patients with head trauma, there was no variance in performance on this test (ie, all subjects scored intact).[8] Therefore, this test may be a poor discriminator for the adult patient with brain damage.

TEST 2: FUNCTIONAL TEST

Description:
Put a pen on the table in front of the patient. Ask him to grasp it. Hold the pen in the air in front of the patient. Ask him to take it from you. Ask the patient to perform other daily activities such as pouring water from a pitcher into a glass or positioning his wheelchair for a transfer.

Scoring:
Subjective.
Intact — patient correctly follows each request without hesitation.
To improve validity, rule out apraxia, poor eye-hand coordination, poor visual acuity, unilateral neglect, and hemianopsia.

Reliability:
In a refined version of this test in a study of adult head trauma patients, 90 percent scored intact, indicating little variance in performance.[8] Additional research should indicate whether the test is appropriate for use with the adult patient with brain damage.

TEST 3: INSTRUCTO CLINIC — DEPTH PERCEPTION TEST[19]

Description:
The patient stands 20 feet away from the testing apparatus, which contains three road signs (stop, yield, and railroad crossing). The patient views four picture sets and is asked to tell which sign is nearest and which is farthest away.

Scoring:
Nonstandardized.
The number of correct responses is calculated and divided into categories of good, satisfactory, and marginal.
To improve validity, rule out aphasia, visual field, and other visual deficits (ie, blurred, double vision) as causes of poor performance.

Treatment of Depth Perception Deficits

Utilizing a Remedial Approach:

1. Apply concepts from the Affolter frame of reference. Provide tactile-kinesthetic guiding during activities. For example, while guiding, have the patient feel the depth, distance and size of his wheelchair before a bed to wheelchair transfer.[12, 20]
2. Utilize computer retraining with software designed specifically for the remediation of depth perception.

Utilizing an Adaptive Approach:

1. Alter the environment to help the patient compensate. For example, place a bright colored tape at the edge of each step of stairs.
2. Have the patient utilize other intact sensory systems rather than visual. For example, utilize tactile sensation in the fingers by having the patient practice pouring by putting his finger near the inside top of a glass to feel when he has poured a full glass.
3. Provide verbal cuing when needed to compensate, especially when safety is an issue.
4. Generally, if the depth perception perception problem is related to decreased binocularity, the patient's cognitive processing skills enable him to compensate. Even though objective testing identifies an impairment, there may be no functional problems (Mary Warren, personal communication). If the depth problem is related to acuity or contrast problems, the therapist identifies the area of function affected and teaches compensation techniques, ie, the use of a cane for stairs (Mary Warren, personal communication).
5. Educate the patient and his family about the depth perception problem and how it will affect function. Areas for which safety is an issue should be highlighted.

Figure Ground Perception

Figure ground perception involves the ability to distinguish the foreground from the background. The "figure" or foreground is the part of the field of perception that is the center of an individual's attention at any given time. Those incoming stimuli which are not the center of attention form a dimly perceived background.[21,22] The separation of figures from background is accomplished by the visual system based on differences in features such as color, luminance, depth, orientation, texture or motion, and temporal information.[23] The difficulty a patient with a figure ground deficit will have visually distinguishing a figure from a competing background will have an impact on his ability to locate objects that are not well defined from the background.[24,25] Higher levels of perception such as figure ground are required to organize the layout of the environment.[26] Therefore, a deficit such as this will adversely affect self-care ability. The patient with a figure ground deficit, for example, may have difficulty finding things in a cluttered drawer or shelf, or finding the sleeve of an all white shirt.

Historically, theories related to the development of figure ground perception assumed that it occurred before any object recognition.[27] It was assumed that visual processes such as figure ground organization depend on variables which are related to the current stimulus and not those from memory which relate to object recognition processes. It was also assumed that object recognition would be impossible unless some prior processes sorted out or reduced the complexity of the problem. One way this is accomplished is through figure ground organization, which differentiates between shaped and shapeless regions in the visual fields.[27]

Some theorists, however, believe that memory does play a role in figure ground perception.[27,28] Recent research indicates that some object or shape recognition occurs before figure ground organization is completed. This shape recognition process has been termed *prefigural recognition processes,* and is an "edged based" recognition process.[27]

Recent research has also highlighted the importance of fixation location and attention to figure ground organization.[10,25,27,29] In a case study of a 69-year-old male with right hemisphere damage, it was discovered that the patient retained figure ground perception despite severe left neglect, even when a stimulus appeared on the left. These researchers conclude that figures are segregated from their background "pre-attentively." Peterson and Gibson take this concept further. They state that not only is there empirical evidence supportive of the relevance of fixation point to figure ground, but also suggest that "the inputs to figure ground organization from fixation location are separate from the inputs from prefigural shape recognition processes."[27]

Evaluation of Figure Ground Perception

TEST 1: AYRES' FIGURE-GROUND TEST

(subtest of the Southern California Sensory Integration Tests)[30]

Description:
This is a published test requiring the patient to select three pictures of objects or geometric forms from a multiple choice plate of six pictures. The three to be selected are to be found in an embedded plate (Figure 6-1). The patient indicates his choice by naming or pointing to the picture or design. He has 1 minute to identify three embedded pictures. The test is discontinued after five errors.

Scoring:
Each correctly identified picture is given a score of 1. The range of possible scores is 0 to 48. This test has been standardized only for children up to the age of 10.11 years. A score of 18 is the mean for 10.11 year olds. The following studies, however, were done with adults. Fifty-six (56) normal adults aged 20-59 were studied, and the results are listed in Table 6-1.

**Figure 6-1. One page
of the Southern
California Figure
Ground Perception
test.**[30]

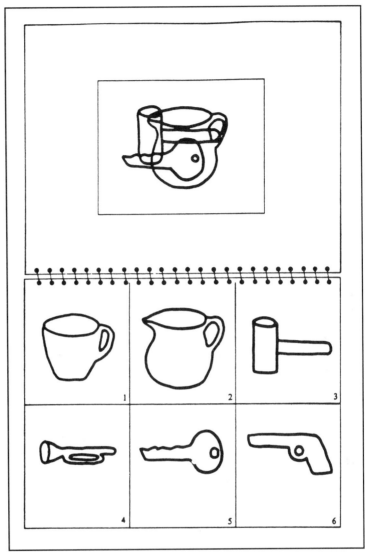

A study was conducted with 100 adult males with the following results:[28] mean score 29.7 (considerably higher than 18.7 norm of 10.3 to 10.11 year olds). Only one male obtained a score of a perfect 48, therefore indicating the test has no ceiling affect. These authors recommend its use with adults.

A study of 124 adult females indicated test results showed a normal distribution and found it to be reliable over time.[22] These authors also recommend its use with adults.

Intact — one standard deviation (±).

Impaired — more than minus 1 standard deviation from the mean.

Severely impaired — more than minus 2 standard deviations from the mean.

Validity:

Rule out poor eyesight, hemianopsia, and dense aphasia. (For mild aphasics who understand gestures, the test may be valid). This test has been found to discriminate between children with and without perceptual deficits ($t=5.19$, $p<0.01$). Its reliability test-retest coefficients of correlation range from $r=0.37$ to 0.52 for children aged 4.0 to 10.11 years.

Table 6-1.

Age	Number of Subjects	Mean Score	One Standard Deviation
20-29	22	31.9	9.7
30-39	12	32.6	8.9
40-49	10	22.8	7.8
50-59	12	23.9	5.7

Reliability:
This test has established inter-rater reliability (r=0.87) on a sample of adult patients with head trauma.[8]
This test requires a high degree of concentration. Therefore, it may not be valid to administer it to patients who show a high degree of distractibility.

TEST 2: OVERLAPPING FIGURES (OF) SUBTEST OF THE L.O.T.C.A.[31]

Description:
This test is based on the classic embedded pictures tests of figure ground perception. The patient is asked to identify six overlapping figures presented on two cards with three figures on each.

Scoring (for the six figures):
1 Point—Patient does not identify any figures, or identifies less than three figures with the aid of the board.
2 Points—Patient identifies three figures with the aid of the board.
3 Points—Patient identifies four figures without the board, or all of the figures with the aid of the board.
4 Points—Patient identifies all of the figures without the board.

Reliability:
Inter-rater reliability with Spearman's rank correlation coefficient between raters ranged from .82 to .97 for the various subtests.

Validity:
The majority of validity and reliability research was conducted on the remaining three subtests. The authors recommend administration of the entire test battery versus utilizing only one or two subtests.

TEST 3: FUNCTIONAL TEST

Description:
The therapist asks the patient to pick out or find an object in view. There are many variations of this test. Here are some examples:
1. While in the patient's bedroom, ask the patient to pick up a white towel or face cloth that you have put on his white sheets.
2. While dressing, ask the patient to find his sleeve, buttonholes, buttons, and bottom of the shirt.
3. While in the kitchen, ask the patient to find objects that are on the counter, or the knife among the unsorted cutlery in the drawer.
4. Ask the patient to sort a pile of shirts into long- and short-sleeved.

Scoring:
Subjective.
Intact—patient does tasks within a reasonable length of time.
To improve validity, rule out poor acuity visual object agnosia and poor comprehension of the directions as reasons for poor performance.

Treatment for Figure Ground Perception

Utilizing a Remedial Approach:

1. Scatter items in front of the patient in a disorganized fashion. Name an object and have the patient point to it. Increase the number of objects in the array as the patient improves.
2. Utilize worksheets, computer programs, etc. which focus on the remediation of figure ground deficits.

Utilizing an Adaptive Approach:

1. Apply concepts from the Dynamic Interactional approach. Identify what strategy for figure ground organization the patient utilizes most effectively (conceptual task characteristics). For example, does he sort a disorganized drawer, or does he utilize systematic scanning for card sorting? If possible, have the patient describe to you how he completed the task. Once it is clear what technique or strategy the patient uses, provide activities in a variety of settings or contexts which allow for application of the identified strategy, ie, the kitchen, grocery store, hardware store, etc. Do not upgrade task requirements until the patient has shown some generalization of learning.
2. Alter the patient's environment as follows:[12]
    a. put only a few things on the night stand
    b. organize drawers, separating articles
    c. arrange the meal tray so that it has only a few items; have the meal in several courses if necessary
    d. mark the wheelchair brakes with red tape so that they will be easier to distinguish from the wheel.
3. To help the patient compensate, teach him cognitive awareness of his deficit; teach him to be very systematic and examine each small area carefully by slowing down and not being impulsive. For example, in the kitchen, have him look and even feel the countertop to find out what objects are on it.
4. Educate the patient and his family regarding the figure-ground deficit and how it will affect function. Train them in the use of compensation techniques such as the need for uncluttered drawers, cabinets, etc.

Spatial Relations

Visual perception is intrinsically spatial.[32] The individual processes descriptions of the external world that inherently contain information about spatial relations within and between objects. When the individual has a consistent point of origin through an established body scheme, continued environmental exploration leads to the perception of areas such as objects and their relationship to the individual or to each other.[12] He can judge distances, distinguish forms and separate objects from a surrounding background. Spatial relations are important to orienting in the environment, recognizing objects and scenes and language.[33] The theoretical basis for the acquisition of spatial relations has recently been explored. Some theorists focus on the importance of spatial attention.[33] They envision the apprehension of spatial relations to involve the coordination of perceptual and conceptual representations of space. The perceptual representations consist of arrays of objects and surfaces, while the conceptual component involves prepositions like above, below, etc.[1] The acquisition process is hypothesized to involve "spatial indexing," which involves the selecting of an object in the perceptual representation and establishing a correspondence between it and a symbol it stands for in the conceptual representation. This process is accomplished through spatial attentional operations. For example, any object can be above something else. Therefore, the number of objects that can serve to relate to the reference object is infinitely large. It is impossible to relate an object to everything, so the relevant relational objects must be selected. Spatial attention is involved in this indexing process as well as in searching for targets that differ from distracters in the spatial relations.[33] These theoretical concepts related to the importance of spatial attention to spatial relations development have recently been supported by clinical research.[33]

Another recent area of focus related to spatial relations acquisition is the existence of two types of spatial relations, that of categorical spatial relations and coordinate spatial relations.[6,32,34-36] Recent research suggests that both the right and left hemispheres can compute both types of spatial relations, but not equally effectively.[32,36] Theorists conceptualize a clear distinction between categorical spatial relations such as above - below, left - right, and on - off, and coordinate spatial relations which specify locations in a way that can be used to guide precise movements. It is further hypothesized that there are distinct subsystems which may encode the two types of spatial relations.[35] Representations are produced by processing subsystems, "with each subsystem corresponding to a set of neurons that work together to transform input into a specific type of output."[6] It is assumed that because categorical and coordinate representations are qualitatively different, separate processing subsystems produce each type of representation.[37]

Evaluation of Spatial Relations

TEST 1: POSITIONING BLOCKS

Description:
The therapist places two small cube blocks in front of the patient and asks him to place one block in various positions in relation to the other block, eg, on top, behind, in front of, to the right, to the left. There is no standardized form of this test. The therapist makes up her own commands.

Scoring:
Subjective.
Intact — patient correctly does each move within a reasonable length of time.
To improve validity, rule out aphasia and apraxia.

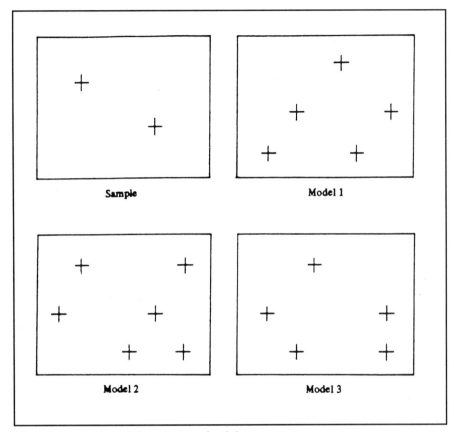

Figure 6-2. Sample and three test cards of the cross test.

Reliability:
In a study of adult patients with head trauma, all 20 subjects scored intact on a variation of this test.[8] Further research should indicate whether this test discriminates well for the adult brain-damaged population.

TEST 2: CROSS TEST[38]

Description:
This test requires the patient to duplicate a small cross on a blank sheet of paper in the same position as it appeared on the stimulus card (Figure 6-2). A blank piece of paper, the sample stimulus card, and a black felt pen are placed in front of the patient, and he is instructed to "Draw two small crosses on this paper in the exact positions that they appear on the card. Be exact." If the patient does not understand, the therapist demonstrates by drawing the crosses for him After the patient does the sample, the transparent score guide is placed over the trial so that the patient can judge the extent of his discrepancies. Then each of the three test cards is presented in turn, with the command: "Now do the same thing with this card. Do not hurry. Be exact."

Scoring:
Nonstandardized. The subject's score is the total number of centimeters of discrepancy between the model and the reproduction. The transparent score guide is placed over the subject's effort, and the distances between the intersection of lines on the model and the

subject's crosses are measured with a centimeter ruler. If there is any doubt as to which cross the patient was attempting to copy, the model closest to his cross should be selected. If a cross is missing from a patient's effort, this should be scored as one-half the width of the page.

Intact — score of 0 to 300.

Impaired — score of 300 to 600.

Severe — score of 600 and above. (Scores adapted from those received by control group study of Pehoski.[39])

To improve validity, rule out motor apraxia, poor eye-hand coordination, unilateral neglect and hemianopsia.

TEST 3: AYRES' SPACE VISUALIZATION TEST

(subtest of Southern California Sensory Integration Tests[30])

Description:

This test uses two formboards, one with an egg-shaped hollow and one with a diamond-shaped hollow, two pegs, four egg-shaped blocks, and four diamond-shaped blocks. The pegs are inserted into the formboards to create different test items. The tests consist of 30 "puzzles," each consisting of one formboard and two blocks, only one of which fits the formboard. The patient is asked to look at the puzzle and choose one of the two blocks. Only then is he allowed to try fitting his choice in the formboard. The test is discontinued after five errors are made.

Scoring:

This test has been standardized only for children. In testing the reliability, Ayres reports the test-retest correlations range from $r=0.28$ to 0.77 for children aged 4.0 to 10.11 years. Using the same scoring method as Ayres, Taylor[39] provides the adult normative data shown in Table 6-2.

Table 6-2

	Age	Number of Subjects	Mean Score	Standard Deviation
Accuracy	50-64	90	56.2	4.5
	65-74	60	56.3	4.5
Time	50-64	90	118.2	50.8
	65-74	60	158.5	74.9

Until a more extensive adult normative study can be done, interpretation of scores is non-standardized.

Intact — one standard deviation.

Impaired — more than minus one standard deviation from the mean.

Validity:

Ayres reported a study in which she administered this test to both right and left hemiplegic adults. The left hemiplegics did better as a group than the right hemiplegics, although the difference was not significant. Because it is generally thought that left hemiplegics do significantly poorer on spatial relations tests, the validity of this test with adults is in some doubt.

Treatment for Spatial Relations

Utilizing a Remedial Approach:

1. Have the patient retrieve objects following verbal requests containing spatial concepts, ie, "Get the brush on top of the dresser behind the bed."
2. Have the patient place a variety of objects in different places around the room. The patient returns to the original spot, visualizes, verbalizes and points to where the objects are in relation to him. Once the patient has localized the objects, he should walk (or wheel) through space to retrieve the objects in sequence.[40]
3. Have the patient practice various tasks for which he must discriminate various spatial relations.
4. Utilize computer retraining with software designed specifically for the remediation of spatial relations deficits.
5. Utilizing an Affolter approach, provide tactile-kinesthetic guiding of the patient to objects and between objects so the patient can receive tactile-kinesthetic input related to object position and distances.

Utilizing an Adaptive Approach:

1. Organize the patient's environment so that necessary items are consistently in the same place. Educate the patient and his family to the patient's spatial relation deficit and the importance of maintaining a consistent environment.
2. Mark areas in drawers, cabinets, etc., where key items are to be stored.

Topographical Disorientation

The patient with topographical disorientation will have difficulty in understanding and remembering relationships of places to one another, so that he may have difficulty in finding his way in space. In order to interact effectively with the environment, we "...require an integrated viewpoint-dependent representation of the world."[41] This viewpoint preserves information about the positions of objects relative to the viewer. To establish this viewpoint, the individual must have adequate visual processing of the dimensions of visual stimuli across the visual fields, adequate depth perception and coding of forms in 3-D, and adequate integration of form information.[41] If these processes are impaired, there can be a decreased ability to recognize visual landmarks and routes. In addition to the visual processes, the individual requires spatial working memory to hold information about where he is and to plan future movements. Adequate attentional processes and stored memories for previously experienced landmarks are also required.

Christianson and Raschko[42] theorize that topographical orientation is accomplished through cognitive mapping.[43] The individual's cognitive map is a mental representation of his surroundings. It is the product of active information seeking, and the means by which one maintains orientation within the environment by recognizing objects and landmarks.

Evaluation of Topographical Disorientation

The test for this deficit is a functional one. If the patient is unable to find his way back to his ward from the treatment room or from occupational therapy to physical therapy after being shown several times, this suggests a topographical disorientation problem. However, one must first rule out a general poor memory problem or mental confusion. Usually topographical disorientation is not seen in isolation from the other problems of spatial relations.

Treatment for Topographical Disorientation
Utilizing an Adaptive Approach:

The following guidelines for environmental adaptations can be utilized to help the patient compensate for this deficit:[42]

1. Identify what spaces or areas can be utilized by the patient as an important landmark. How or with what type of marker should the space be identified, and where should such identification be located?

2. Provide landmarks such as pictures or objects that provide "...cues that give one knowledge or feeling of where one is in a particular place,"[42] eg, murals, paintings.

3. Landmark designs and signs should be clear and realistic. Utilize high contrast, ie, colors that contrast with the wall for patients with visual deficits.

4. Any signs or landmarks placed for the patient in a wheelchair should have the lower edge placed at 54" high and to the latch side of the door.

5. Signs should have contrast between the lettering and background and should avoid busy patterns.

6. Specific areas where signs facilitate topographical orientation are entries and exits, bathrooms and eating areas.

References

1. Jolicoeur P, Ullman S, Mackay M. Curve tracing: A possible basic operation in the perception of spatial relations. *Memory & Cogn.* 1986;14(2):129-140.
2. Gulyas B, Heywood CA, Popplewell DA, Roland PE, Cowey A. Visual form discrimination from color or motion cues: Functional anatomy by positron emission tomography. *Proc. Natl. Acad. Science.* Oct 1994;91:9965-9969.
3. Livingstone MS, Hubel DH. Psychophysical evidence for separate channels for the perception of form, color, movement, and depth. *J of Neuroscience.* 1987;7(11):3416-3468.
4. Marsolek CJ. Abstract visual-form representations in the left cerebral hemisphere. *J Exper Psych Hum Percept Perform.* 1995;21(2):375-386.
5. Rock I, DiVita J, Barbeito R. The effect on form perception of change of orientation in the third dimension. *J Exper Psych Human Percept Perform.* Aug 1991;7(4):719-732.
6. Kosslyn S, Chabris CF, Marsolek CJ, Koenig O. Categorical versus coordinate spatial relations: Computational analyses and computer simulations. *J Exp Psych: Hum Percept Perform.* 1992;18(2):562-577.
7. Zoltan B, Jabri J, Panikoff L, Ryckman D. *Perceptual Motor Evaluation for Head Injured and Other Neurologically Impaired Adults.* San Jose, California. Santa Clara Valley Medical Center, Occupational Therapy Department; 1983.

8. Baum B. The establishment of reliability and validity of a perceptual evaluation on a sample of adult head trauma patients. Thesis, University of Southern California, December 1981.

9. Dannenbaum RM, Jones LA. The assessment and treatment of patients who have sensory loss following cortical lesions. *J of Hand Therapy*. April-June 1993:130-138.

10. Rock I, Mitchener K. Further evidence of failure of reversal of ambiguous figures by uninformed subjects. *Perception*. 1992;21:39-45.

11. Rizzo M. Astereopsis. In: Boller F, Grafman J (eds). *Handbook of Neuropsychology* (Vol. 2) . Amsterdam, Elsevier Science Pubs.; 1989.

12. Zoltan B. Remediation of visual-perceptual and perceptual-motor deficits. In: Rosenthal M, Griffith ER, Bond MR, Miller JD (eds.). *Rehabilitation of the Adult and Child with Traumatic Brain Injury*. Philadelphia, FA Davis Co.; 1990.

13. Neger RE. The evaluation of diplopia in head trauma. *J Head Trauma Rehabil*. 1989;4(2):27-34.

14. Newcombe F, Ratcliff G. Disorders of visuospatial analysis. In: Boller F, Grafman J (eds). *Handbook of Neuropsychology* (Vol. 2). Amsterdam, Elsevier Science Pubs.; 1989.

15. Westheimer G, Levi DM. Depth attraction and repulsion of disparate foveal stimuli. *Vision Res*. 1987;27(8):1361-1368.

16. Nakayama K, Shimojo S. Da Vinci stereopsis: Depth and subjective occluding contours from unpaired image points. *Vision Res*. 1990;30(11):1811-1825.

17. Brown JM, Weisstein N. A spatial frequency effect on perceived depth. *Percept & Psychophys*. 1988;44(2):157-166.

18. Goldberg ME, Colby CL. The neurophysiology of spatial vision. In: Boller F, Grafman J. (eds). *Handbook of Neuropsychology* (Vol. 2). Amsterdam, Elsevier Science Pubs.; 1989.

19. *Instructo-Clinic—A Psychophysical Testing Apparatus*. Bumpa-Tel, Inc., P.O. Box 611, Cape Cir., Missouri 63701.

20. Affolter FD. *Perception, Interaction and Language; Interaction of Daily Living: The Root of Development*. Berlin, Springer-Verlag Co.; 1987.

21. Craine J. The retraining of frontal lobe dysfunction. In: Trexler LE. (ed.). *Cognitive Rehabilitation: Conceptualization and Intervention*. New York, Plenum Press; 1982.

22. Petersen P, Goar D, Van Deusen J. Performance of female adults on the Southern California Visual Figure-Ground Perception Test. *Amer J Occup Ther*. 1985;39(8):525-530.

23. Fahle M. Figure-ground discrimination from temporal information. *Proc R Soc Lond B Biol Sci*. 1993;254(1341):199-203.

24. Capitani E, Della Sala S, Lucchelli F, Soave P, Spinnler H. Perceptual attention in aging and dementia measured by Gottschaldt's Hidden Figure Test. *J of Gerontology: Psychological Sciences*. 1988;43(6):157-163.

25. Driver J, Baylis GC, Rafal RD. Preserved figure-ground segregation and symmetry perception in visual neglect. *Nature*. 1992;360:73-75.

26. Bernspang B, Asplund K, Eriksson S, Fugl-Meyer AR. Motor and perceptual impairments in acute stroke patients: Effects on self-care ability. *Stroke*. 1987;18(6):1081-1086.

27. Peterson MA and Gibson BS. Object recognition contributions to figure-ground organization: Operations on outlines and subjective contours. *Perc & Psych*. 1994;56(5):551-564.

28. Petersen P, Wikoff RL. The performance of adult males on the Southern California Figure-Ground Visual Perception Test. *Amer J Occup Ther*. 1983;37(8):554-560.

29. Lagreze WD, Meigen T, Bach M. Asymmetries in texture perception. *Ger J Ophthalmol*. 1994;3(4-5):220-223.

30. Ayres AJ. S*outhern California Sensory Integration Tests*. Los Angeles, Western Psychological Services; 1972.

31. Itzkovich M, Arerback S, Belazar. *Lowenstein Occupational Therapy Cognitive Assessment*. Maddack Inc., Pequanock, NJ.

32. Sergent J. Judgments of relative position and distance on representations of spatial relations. *J Exp Psych: Hum Percept Perform*. 1991;91(3):762-780.

33. Logan GD. Spatial attention and the apprehension of spatial relations. *J Exper Psych: Hum Percept Perform*. 1994;20(5):1015-1036.

34. Hoyer WJ, Rybash JM. Age and visual field differences in computing visual-spatial relations. *Psych & Aging.* 1992;7(3):339-342.
35. Jacobs RA and Kosslyn SM. Encoding shape and spatial relations: The role of receptive field size in coordinating complementary representations. *Cogn Science.* 1994;18:361-386.
36. Kosslyn SM, Koenig O, Barrett A, Backer-Cave C, Tang J, Gabrieli JDE. Evidence for two types of spatial representations: Hemispheric specialization for categorical and coordinate relations. *J Exp Psych: Hum Percept Perform.* 1989;15(4):723-735.
37. Kosslyn SM, Chabris CF, Jacobs RA, Marsolek CJ, Koenig O. On computational evidence for different types of spatial relations encoding: Reply to Cook et al. (1995). *J Exp Psych: Hum Percept Perform.* 1995;21(2):423-431.
38. Pehoski C. Analysis of perceptual dysfunction and dressing in adult hemiplegics. Thesis, Sargent College, Boston University; 1970.
39. Taylor MM. Analysis of dysfunction in the left hemiplegia following stroke. *Am J Occup Ther.* 1968;22:512-520.
40. Bouska MJ, Kauffman NA, Marcus SE. Disorders of the visual perceptual system, In: Umphred DA (ed). *Neurological Rehabilitation (2nd edition).* St. Louis, CV Mosby Co.; 1990.
41. Riddoch MJ, Humphreys GW. Finding the way around topograghical impairments. In: Brown W (ed.). *Neuropsychology of Visual Impairments.* New Jersey, Lawrence Erlbaum Assoc.; 1989.
42. Christenson MA, Raschko B. Environmental cognition and age-related sensory change. *Occup Ther Pract.* 1989;1(1):28-35.
43. Cohen M, GrossWasser Z, Banchadske R, Appel A. Convergence insufficiency in brain-injured patients, *Brain Injury.* 1989;3(2):187-191.

CHAPTER 7

Agnosia

Agnosia, the area of deficits that deals with the patient's lack of recognition of familiar objects perceived by the senses, occurs frequently in patients who have sustained a C.V.A. or T.B.I. It may involve a disturbance in one or all of the following sensory modes—visual, tactile, proprioceptive, and auditory—or may involve additional problems in body scheme, such as somatognosia or anosognosia.

Visual Agnosia

The theoretical basis of visual agnosia includes descriptions of both a perceptive and associative agnosia. A perceptive agnosia is believed to be the result of a disordered perception, even though primary visual functions are present.[1,2] There is a distortion of the stimulus at the sensory-perceptual levels which causes a failure to recognize visually presented objects. The patient cannot name, copy or recognize visually presented objects but can readily identify the object with tactile or auditory cues.[1]

Associative visual agnosia is the result of a disordered association. The patient with associative visual agnosia is unable to recognize familiar objects despite adequate perception.[2] These patients can copy figures or written material and name objects from verbal definitions.[1,3] Many patients with visual associative agnosia do well on the majority of visual tests, such as block designs or embedded pictures. These remaining skills suggest that they have "retained the conceptual and linguistic abilities needed to demonstrate recognition."[3]

The lesion sites and mechanisms which cause aperceptive and associative visual agnosia remain controversial. The process or requirements of object recognition, however, are succinctly described by Ellis and Young as follows:

> We can think of object recognition as requiring that viewer-centered and object-centered representations of seen objects are matched to stored descriptions of known objects, object recognition units, which then allow access to semantic representations (spoken name).[4]

Functional impairments, which can occur as the result of visual agnosia, are diverse and potentially devastating to the patient. The patient can fail to recognize close relatives or precious possessions. The following sections outline the major types of visual agnosia that the patient may exhibit.

Visual Object Agnosia

As previously described, visual object agnosia is the inability to recognize objects presented visually, although the primary visual skills such as acuity are intact.

Evaluation of Visual Object Agnosia

TEST 1: OBJECT RECOGNITION[5]

Description:
Several common objects such as a key, comb, toothbrush, or coins are placed in front of the patient. Ask the patient to pick up the object that is named, or demonstrate or describe its functional use.

Scoring:
The examiner may assume the object is recognized if any of the following occurs:
• the patient names, describes or demonstrates the use of an object, or
• selects it from among a group of objects as it is named by the examiner.

TEST 2: L.O.T.C.A.—VISUAL IDENTIFICATION OF OBJECTS[6]

Description:
The visual identification subtest (VO) is one of several subtests of the L.O.T.C.A. The remaining subtests are described in the section on orientation in Chapter 8.

Procedure:
The patient is shown eight cards of illustrated everyday objects: chair, teapot, watch, key, shoe, bicycle, scissors, glasses. The patient is asked to name each object.

If the patient is not able to name the objects because of expressive problems (eg, expressive or amnestic aphasia, or severe disarthria), he is shown two boards with four objects presented on each. The examiner asks the patient, "Where is a chair?," "Where is a watch?" etc. This procedure is used for each of the eight objects.

If patient has receptive/expressive problems (eg, global or receptive/expressive aphasia), the examiner should show him two boards with four similar objects presented on each. The patient has to match the target objects with the similar one on the boards. If the patient is unable to identify similar objects, the examiner presents him the two boards with the identical objects. The patient has to do an exact matching.

Scoring:
1 point — The patient identifies only a few objects by exact matching (less than four).
2 points — The patient identifies five to eight objects by exact matching.
3 points — The patient identifies at least four objects by naming, understanding, or similar matching (4-7).
4 points — The patient identifies all the objects by naming, understanding, or similar matching.

Reliability:
Interrater reliability with Spearman's rank correlation coefficient for subtests ranged from .82 to .97. Internal consistency reliability through Cronback's alpha coefficient was calculated at .87 for the five subtests of perception which includes object identification. The authors caution, however, that all parts of the battery should be given due to correlation coefficients ranging from .40 to .80 among the subtests.

Validity:
The authors state the Wilcoxin two-sample test was used to compare the control and patient group. Results state the subtests, except the object identification subtest, differentiated at the .0001 level of significance. I was unable to find the measure for the object identification subtest.

Treatment of Visual Object Agnosia

Utilizing a Remedial Approach:

1. Have the patient practice identifying objects which are needed for functional independence.
2. Apply concepts from the Affolter approach. Provide nonverbal, tactile-kinesthetic guiding through an activity. "After the activity, take some of the tools used in the task and follow up the guided activity with naming the items that were used. Ask the patient to recreate the steps in the task, either with words, or with picture identification, sequencing cards, etc." (personal communication, Karen Bonfils).

Utilizing an Adaptive Approach:

1. Encourage the patient to manipulate the object with simultaneous visual and verbal input.[5] Use intact sensory modalities.[8]
2. Provide labels for objects as necessary to maximize independence.

Prosopagnosia

An individual's face tells us about areas such as gender, age, race and emotion. It also conveys information about the individual's physical uniqueness by the particular arrangement of specific features. These features provide clues to the person's identity.[4]

Prosopagnosia is a neurologically based deficit characterized by the inability to identify a known individual by his face. This inability is seen in the absence of severe sensory, intellectual and visual impairments.[1,4,9,10] The patient knows he is looking at a face but cannot say to whom the face belongs.

The inability to recognize familiar faces is associated with a lesion to the right posterior hemisphere.[9,10] It is rarely seen in isolation and often associated with object agnosia.[4] Some clinicians believe the problem is perceptual in nature, while others believe it is primarily due to decreased memory.[4,9] Still others believe it is not due to perceptual or memory loss but to an impairment of the activation step which does not take place, or takes place inefficiently.[11] Two distinct categories of patients have been identified: 1) patients who cannot perceive faces, which is related to a problem with structural encoding, and 2) patients who appear to have relatively intact perceptual abilities but cannot recognize or in some way process the faces they seem to perceive.[4,10]

Evaluation of Prosopagnosia

TEST 1: FUNCTIONAL EVALUATION

Although there are many tests of facial matching and identification, a functional evaluation is recommended.

Procedure:
Therapist has the patient identify key members of the family, friends and coworkers. Identification is made through photographs, and whenever possible, the actual person.

Scoring:
Individuals who could not be identified through facial recognition are identified.

Treatment of Prosopagnosia

Utilizing a Remedial Approach:

1. Provide face matching and progressive face sequence tasks.

Utilizing an Adaptive Approach:

1. Provide pictures with names, pictures of the unrecognized individual(s) in different settings at different angles, and with other people the patient is able to recognize.
2. Help the patient associate the individual's face with other features and characteristics such as voice, haircut, manner of walk, height, clothes, etc.
3. Review with the patient a video with the individual in which he is talking.

Simultagnosia

Simultagnosia is the inability to recognize a compound visual array.[4] These patients are unable to perceive more than one thing at a time and the amount of time necessary to distinguish between two perceptual acts is excessively long. They are unable to recognize the abstract meaning of a whole stimulus array even though the details are correctly perceived. They are able to describe specific elements of a complex stimulus, but cannot integrate these elements to achieve recognition of the picture.

Some clinicians believe simultagnosia is partly caused by defective short-term visual memory loss.[9] Others have observed that although these patients have normal visual field on parametric testing, they will shrink to narrow vision when concentrating on the visual environment.

In summary, simultagnosia is a disorder which involves impairment in interpreting a visual stimulus as a whole. It seems to result from an extreme reduction in visual span of apprehension.[12] Given a whole picture, the patient absorbs only one aspect or part at a time. For instance, a patient could point out individual letters or features, but cannot give an accurate account of the whole word.[12]

Color Agnosia

Color agnosia is the inability to recognize colors such that the patient cannot pick out a color or name a color on command.[13] This patient should be able to say whether two colors are the same or different if visual sensation is still intact. Color agnosia appears to occur more commonly after left hemisphere lesions.

Metamorphopsia

Metamorphopsia is a visual distortion of objects, although the object may be recognized accurately. For instance, a chair may appear larger or smaller than it actually is.

Visual Spatial Agnosia

Visual spatial agnosia is a deficit in perceiving spatial relationships between objects or between objects and self, independently of visual object agnosia. Visual spatial agnosia can include the following difficulties:

1. Difficulty with spatial relations.
2. Difficulty in judging distances such that the patient may go to sit in a chair and misjudge so that he misses the chair.
3. Difficulty in depth perception such that the patient may continue pouring water into a glass after it is filled.

Topographagnosia

Topographagnosia is an impairment in the interpretation of maps, house plans, etc.[1] The patient can perform normally in real situations but cannot place himself on a map.[1] These patients are unable to draw a plan of their house or identify rooms on a plan that is drawn for them.

Environmental Agnosia

Patients with environmental agnosia will get lost in familiar places. These patients can read maps and house plans well, but cannot find their way even in familiar places.[1]

Patients may have one type of problem without the others.

Tactile Agnosia

Tactile agnosia is a modality specific disorder which is evidenced by an inability to recognize objects tactually, although tactile, thermal, and proprioceptive functions are still intact.[14,15] The patient cannot associate the retrieved tactile image with other sensory images. He cannot recognize the object, although able to recognize the tactile qualities.

Tactile agnosia, often called astereognosis, is believed by some to be a high level perceptual disorder that can occur from a failure to "integrate accurately acquired somesthetic features into a haptic mental image which can then be manipulated."[15] In a study of C.V.A. patients, Reed and Casselli found that tactile agnosia can occur with high level faulty perceptual processes, but that the ability to associate tactually defined objects and object parts can be preserved.[15]

Stereognosis requires the integration of information related to the temperature, texture, weight and contour of an object, and involves both the cutaneous and proprioceptive (muscle and joint receptors) sensory systems.[16] The identification of objects through touch and somesthetic sensations is accomplished by:

1. Primary identification through recognition of texture, form, etc.
2. Secondary recognition of the significance of the object.[14]

There are four types of information processing in the tactile recognition system:[14]

1. Ahylognosia—disturbance in the ability to discriminate materials
2. Amorphagnosia—disturbance in the ability to discriminate forms
3. Tactile agnosia—inability to recognize familiar objects
4. Tactile aphasia—inability to name tactually identified objects in the absence of aphasic anomia

Tactile agnosia can occur with or without the other deficits of the tactile recognition system.

Evaluation of Tactile Agnosia

TEST 1: STEREOGNOSIS[17-19]

Description:
Tell the patient, "I am going to put a form like one of these in your hand so that you can feel it for a little while. Then I'll show you all the forms and you can show me the one that was in your hand." Demonstrate by putting one of the objects in the patient's hand and having him feel it. Then put it back in the tray and have him show you which object he felt. Occlude the patient's vision by having him close his eyes, shield them with a file folder, or use a box like the one described in Test 1 under Finger Agnosia. Be sure that the patient does not drop objects onto the table and get auditory cues, eg, by running a finger along teeth of comb. Common objects often used for this test are a ball, spoon, pencil, key, penny, ring, button, block, and scissors. Test each hand alternately.

Scoring:
Nonstandardized.
Intact - patient correctly identifies all objects within a reasonable length of time. Normal subjects can name a familiar object within five seconds of contact.[16] The time required for recognition should be recorded, as well as whether the patient can identify the object.[19]
To improve validity, rule out impaired tactile sensation and paresis in the affected hand so that the patient cannot feel or move the object around to feel its shape. Rule out impaired sensation in the nonaffected hand.

TEST 2: AYRES' MANUAL FORM PERCEPTION
(subtest of Southern California Sensory Integration Tests)[20]

Description:
Procedure is the same as in Test 1. Objects used are ten plastic geometric forms, eg, oval, triangle, circle, star, square, hexagon, octagon, diamond, cross, and trapezoid. The object is placed in the patient's hand while his vision is occluded by a file folder shield. The patient

is asked to identify the object he is feeling from twelve geometric forms printed on a piece of cardboard placed before him. Hands are tested alternately. Bilateral manipulation of a form is not allowed.

Scoring:
This test has been standardized for children aged 4.0 to 8.11 years. In testing reliability, Ayres reports that the test-retest correlations range from r=0.20 to 0.64. Scoring for adults is nonstandardized.
Intact—patient correctly identifies all ten forms within a reasonable length of time.
To improve validity, rule out impaired tactile sensation and paresis of the affected hand and impaired sensation of the nonaffected hand.

TEST 3: MORPHOGNOSIS

Description:
Same as test for stereognosis except that one uses geometric shapes cut out of stiff paper, only 1/32 inch thick, instead of three-dimensional objects. Common shapes used are a diamond, circle, triangle, octagon, square, and egg shape.

Scoring:
Nonstandardized.
Intact—patient correctly identifies all shapes within a reasonable length of time.
To improve validity, rule out lack of tactile sensation and paresis of the affected hand and impaired sensation of the nonaffected hand.

TEST 4: AHYLOGNOSIS

Description:
Same as test for stereognosis except that one uses materials of different textures. Some common materials used are rough and fine sandpaper, silk, plastic wrap, terry cloth, and corduroy.

Scoring:
Nonstandardized.
Intact—patient correctly identifies all textures within a reasonable length of time.
To improve validity, rule out impaired tactile sensation and paresis of the affected hand and impaired sensation of the nonaffected hand.

Treatment of Tactile Agnosia

Utilizing a Remedial Approach:

1. Based on the belief that the brain has potential for recovery of sensory function through reorganization, provide sensory retraining as follows:[16]

    a.   establish some appreciation of sensory inputs from the receptors in the fingertips.

    stage 1: a stimulus such as hooked Velcro is moved along the fingertips

    stage 2: when the patient can appreciate the moving stimulus, then progress to the appreciation of stationary tactile inputs which is required for holding tasks.

Utilizing an Adaptive Approach:

1.   Provide the following to help the patient compensate:[21]

a. increase the patient's awareness of the problem, especially how it will affect function and personal safety, eg, kitchen.

b. place emphasis on sensory tasks which the patient can do at the start and finish of each treatment session.

c. choose sensory tasks that will interest the patient and which will lead to sufficient successes and failures to promote learning.

d. utilize other senses such as vision and use of the good hand to teach tactics of perception.

e. train the patient to focus on the specific properties of the object, ie, contour, texture, or temperature.[16]

2. Utilizing the concept that object recognition is accomplished through the interaction of top-down and bottom-up processing, facilitate object recognition through access of associated sorted personal memories.[15] In other words, provide objects for which the patient can draw on past experience with the object and its features.

Auditory Agnosia

Auditory agnosia is the inability to recognize differences in sounds, including both word and nonword sounds. For example, a patient may not be able to differentiate between the sound of a car engine running and the sound of a vacuum cleaner.

Evaluation and Treatment of Auditory Agnosia

Evaluation and treatment for auditory agnosia are usually done by the speech therapist.

Apractognosia

Apractognosia consists of several different apraxic and agnostic syndromes, all centering mainly around a lack of perspective.[13] Resulting from a lesion in the nondominant hemisphere, apractognosia may include one or all of the following:

1. Body scheme problems
   a. denial of left hemiplegia
   b. lack of awareness of left half of body or space
   c. feelings of strangeness
   d. right-left disorientation for both personal and extrapersonal space
2. Apraxia for dressing
   a. faulty application of clothes to the body because the patient cannot understand the relationship of the clothes to the body
   b. faulty right-left manipulations used in tying a tie or a shoe
3. Constructional apraxia due to lack of perspective
4. Unilateral spatial agnosia
   a. loss of conception of topographical relationships such that the patient could no longer conceive that the bathroom is down the hall to the left of his room

b. disturbances of orientation such that the patient does not know where he is

c. loss of topographical memory such that the patient has forgotten his familiar routes from one place to another

d. visual coordinate problems such that the patient has difficulty perceiving the vertical and horizontal correctly

Evaluation and Treatment for Apractognosia

Evaluation and treatment for the apractognosia syndrome may be found under the corresponding apraxic and agnostic deficits on the following pages:

1. Body scheme disorders:
   a. anosognosia, page 82
   b. unilateral neglect, page 80
   c. right-left disorientation, page 83
2. Dressing apraxia, page 67
3. Constructional apraxia for the nondominant hemisphere, page 61
4. Visual spatial agnosia
   a. topographical discrimination, page 103 and also under Spatial Relations Syndrome, page 103

Agnosias Related to Body Scheme Disorders

1. Somatognosia: See this description under Body Scheme Disorders, page 74
2. Anosognosia: See this description under Body Scheme Disorders, page 81
3. Finger Agnosia: See this description under Body Scheme Disorders, page 84

References

1. Benson DF. Disorders of Visual Gnosis. In: Brown JW (ed.). *Neuropsychology of Visual Perception.* New Jersey, Lawrence Erlbaum Assoc.; 1989.
2. Schnider A, Benson F, Scharre W. Visual agnosia and optic aphasia: Are they anatomically distinct? *Cortex.* 1994;30:440-457.
3. Feinberg TE, Schindler RL, Ochoa E, Kwan P, Farah MP. Associative visual agnosia and alexia without prosognosia. *Cortex.* 1994;30:395-412.
4. Ellis AW, Young AW. *Human Cognitive Neuropsychology.* Hillsdale, New Jersey, Lawrence Erlbaum Assoc.; 1988.
5. Bouska MJ, Kauffman NA, Marcus SE. Disorders of the visual perceptual system. In: Umphred DA (ed). *Neurological Rehabilitation* (2nd edition). St. Louis, CV Mosby Co.; 1990.
6. Itzkovich M, Arerback S, Belazar. *Lowenstein Occupational Therapy Cognitive Assessment.* Maddack Inc., Pequanock, NJ.
7. Warrington E, James M. *The Visual Object and Space Perception Battery.* Thames Valley Test Co., Bury St. Edmunds; 1991.
8. Rubio KB, Van Deusen J. Relation of perceptual and body image dysfunction to activities of daily living of persons after stroke. *Amer J of Occup Ther.* 1995;49(6):551-559.
9. Parker RS. *Traumatic Brain Injury and Neuropsychological Impairment.* New York, Springer-Verlag; 1990.
10. Sergent J and Villemure JG. *Prosopagnosia in a Right Hemispherectomized Patient.* Oxford University Press; 1989.

11. Tranel D, Damasio AR. Knowledge without awareness: An autonomic index of facial recognition by prosopagnosics. *Science*. June 1985;228:1453-1454.
12. Warington E, Rabin P. Visual span of apprehension in patients with unilateral cerebral lesions. *Quart J Exp Psychol*. 1971;23:423-431.
13. Hecaen H, Penfield W, Bertrand C, Malmo R. The syndrome of apractognosis due to lesions of the minor cerebral hemisphere. *Arch Neurol Psychiat*. 1956;75:400-434.
14. Endo K, Miyasaka M, Makishkta H, Yanagisawa N, Susishita M. Tactile agnosia and tactile aphasia: Symptomatological and anatomical differences. *Cortex*. 1992;28:445-469.
15. Reed C, Caselli RJ. The nature of tactile agnosia: A case study. *Neuropsychologia*. 1994;32(5):527-539.
16. Dannenbaum RM, Jones LA. The assessment and treatment of patients who have sensory loss following cortical lesions. *J of Hand Therapy*. April-June 1993:130-138.
17. Cook EA, Thigpen R. Identification and management of cognitive and perceptual deficits in the rehabilitation patient. *Rehabilitation Nursing*. Sept/Oct 1993; 18(5): 3110-3113.
18. Deitz JC, Tovar VS, Thorn DW, Beeman C. The test of orientation for rehabilitation patients: inter-rater reliability. *Amer J of Occup Therapy*. 1990;44(9):784-790.
19. Robertson SL, Jones LA. Tactile sensory impairments and prehensile function in subjects with left hemisphere cerebral lesions. *Arch Phys Med Rehabil*. 1994;75:1108-1117.
20. Ayres AJ. *Southern California Sensory Integration Tests*. Los Angeles, Western Psychological Services; 1972.
21. Fox JVD. Effect of cutaneous stimulation on performance of hemiplegic adults on selected tests of perception. Thesis, University of Southern California; 1963.

CHAPTER 8

Orientation, Attention and Memory

Orientation

The T.B.I. or C.V.A. patient who is disoriented is unsure of time, person or place. These difficulties will cause problems in orienting oneself in space with reference to distance and to objects.[1] There can be an altered sense of time and the patient will often get lost. Some aspects of disorientation may indicate a problem with retrograde memory loss, while others reflect problems with new learning or anterograde memory.[2]

Orientation to person, for example, is a retrograde memory loss for autobiographical information. The patient may also not remember his or her previous social role.[3] Orientation to date, place and present circumstances, on the other hand, requires the ability to take in, store and later recall new information. One study of 80 T.B.I. patients indicated a quicker recovery of orientation to person. The authors hypothesized that orientation to place and time may be more vulnerable because of this dependency on the retention of new information.[4] The patient must also be able to monitor and store his or her internal map which serves to assist in self-locating within the environment. Deitz et al[3] outline nine characteristics common to orientation loss as follows:

1. Orientation may be reflected verbally or behaviorally.
2. Disorientation may be temporary or long-lasting.
3. Orientation tends to be viewed as an all-or-none phenomenon, although criteria vary from clinician to clinician.
4. Some domains of orientation appear more resistant to breakdown than others, with the dimension of time appearing to be the most vulnerable.
5. The most common sequence of recovery of orientation following brain injury is person, place and time.
6. Temporal orientation is multidimensional.
7. Disorientation is likely to be associated with memory impairment.
8. Orientation is vulnerable to the effects of brain injury.
9. When long-lasting, disorientation requires attention because it may constitute an important obstacle to management and rehabilitation.

Evaluation of Orientation

TEST 1: TEST OF ORIENTATION FOR REHABILITATION PATIENTS (TORP)[3]*

Description:
The TORP contains 46 items and measures orientation to person and personal situation, place, time, schedule, and temporal continuity. It requires only verbal response and is not appropriate for use with severely aphasic patients, but can be adapted for nonverbal patients. Each test item is written both as an open-ended question and as an auditory recognition task. The recognition task is used only if the patient is unable to respond or responds incorrectly to the open-ended task.

Scoring:
2.00 — answers open ended question
1.00 — responds to auditory recognition task
0.00 — patient does not respond correctly

Reliability:
Test-retest reliability was established with a TBI group with correlations as follows:
.86 person and personal situation
.92 place
.83 time
.72 schedule
.85 temporal continuity
.95 total test
Inter-rater reliability was established through intraclass correlations ranging from .94 to .99.

Validity:
Content validity was established by a panel of expert judges through a specific item rating form relative to each of the five domains. Data were analyzed at the item and domain level. For all five domains, coefficient of agreement (Lu's coefficient) were statistically significant beyond the .05 level.
Two items are provided as examples.

Person and Personal Situation:
"What is your first name?"

Recognition:
"Is your first name …?"

Sam	Roy	George	or	(Correct)	/	Mike
or						
Sheila	Amy	Judy	or	(Correct)	/	Harriet

Accept: Correct first name or nickname.

"In what kind of place were you staying right before you came to this (hospital/rehabilitation center)?"

Place:
"What kind of place is this room in?"

---

*Reproduced with permission from Therapy Skill Builders/Communication Skill Builders, 3830 E. Bellevue, PO Box 42050, Tucson, AZ 85733.

Recognition: *Is this room in…?*
your home   a bank   a hotel   or   (Correct)

Accept: Correct identification of type of place (ie, hospital, rehabilitation center). If patient gives more specific response such as "occupational therapy department," the examiner should rephrase the question. For example, the examiner might then ask, *"What kind of place is the occupational therapy department in?"*

TEST 2: LOWENSTEIN OCCUPATIONAL THERAPY COGNITIVE ASSESSMENT (L.O.T.C.A.) ORIENTATION SUBTEST[5]*

Description:
The orientation subtest contains two items and is one of four subtests of the L.O.T.C.A. The other areas are perception, visuomotor organization and thinking operations. Clinical observation of attention and concentration are also included.

Procedure:
Orientation for Place (ORP)
Patient is asked where he or she is now, ie, the name of the hospital and the name of the city in which it is located.
The examiner asks the patient the following questions:
"Where are you now?"
"Where is it located?"
"Where do you live? What is your exact address?"
"Name a city that is located near your home address."
Orientation for Time (ORT)
The examiner asks the patient the following questions:
"What day is today? What month? What year?"
"What is the hour now?"
"How long have you been hospitalized?"
Orientation comments:
Total disorientation for place and time indicates a confusional state. Generally, ORP improves before ORT.

Scoring:
Scoring is on a scale of 1 (low) to 4 (high).
For the first item, if the patient answers all of the questions correctly, he gets 2 points. For partial performance or no performance, he gets 1 point. For the other two items, the patient receives 1 point for each correct answer.
Minimal performance—1
Maximal performance—4

Reliability:
Inter-rater reliability with Spearman's rank correlation coefficient between raters ranged from .82 to .97 for the various subtests.

Validity:
The majority of validity and reliability research was conducted on the remaining three sub-

---

*Reproduced with permission from Maddak, Inc., 6 Industrial Road, Pequannock, NJ 07440.

tests. The authors recommend administration of the entire test battery versus utilizing only one or two subtests.

Treatment for Orientation

Utilizing a Remedial Approach:

1. Have the patient participate in a daily orientation group. Group sessions should provide a structured setting for repetitive and consistent management of topics involved.[6] When designing and setting up the group, focus on member selections, meeting frequency, meeting place, treatment, media and staff, and family education.
2. Provide daily individual reality orientation in a consistent, structured manner for areas of patient disorientation.

Utilizing an Adaptive Approach:

1. Provide external orientation aids such as labeled pictures of family members, friends, pets, etc. Watches, large calendars, and orientation boards are also helpful.
2. Rotate personal items brought from home, ie, favorite possessions, radio, TV.[6]
3. The patient's daily routine should be as organized and consistent as possible. This is also true of the patient's room and personal environment.
4. Educate the patient's family regarding the patient's disorientation and explain to them the importance of a consistent daily routine and stable, consistent personal environment.

Attention

Attention is often used as a "catch all" term to describe many aspects of behavior. It is an active process that helps to determine which sensations and experiences are alerting and relevant to the individual. Without attention, there can be no further information processing.[7] By deciding what we pay attention to, we decide what information is transferred from sensory memory to meaningful images that can be stored. Attention needs to be directed to a sensory input before any interpretation can take place.[8] Concentration deficits can prevent adequate attending which in turn can affect memory. Effort and concentration are required for the processing of new information.

Historically, most theories related to attention equated it with information processing.[9] Subsequently, the concept of selectivity was developed. In other words, a target stimulus received priority over a non-target stimulus. This selectivity allows the individual to respond to a specific event and inhibit all simultaneous events.

Attentional abilities are inter-related to a number of cognitive systems and therefore should be viewed as a component of interconnected abilities.[10] It is a common occurrence that as attentional disorders recover, many information processing and cognitive deficits become apparent.[11] Parente[7] incorporates this concept of interconnected abilities in his seven stage model of attention training. The model incorporates seven related skills as follows:

1. Basic arousal
2. Simple orientation to a visual/auditory stimulus
3. Attention with discrimination
4. Concentration and mental control
5. Distracted attention
6. Attention with immediate memory
7. Interference resistance training

There are two types of information processing that are related to attention: automatic and controlled processing. Controlled processing is utilized when new information is being considered. Automatic processing, on the other hand, occurs at a subcortical level.[12] Many clinicians are already aware of the behavior patients exhibit relative to these two types of processing. For example, the patient who has sustained a C.V.A. or T.B.I. requires conscious attention to complete even the simplest tasks.[12] Two disorders, focused attentional deficit and divided attentional deficit, are related to these processing concepts and can occur after a C.V.A. or T.B.I.

Toglia[13] views attention not as separate subskills that form a hierarchy, but rather analyzes attentional function/dysfunction in relation to the interaction of task characteristics, environment and the individual. The complexity or familiarity of a given task, for example, will determine the extent to which particular aspects of attention are required.[13] The demands placed on each aspect of attention can differ depending on the situation. During one task, a patient may exhibit good selective attention and poor attentional flexibility, while with a different task, the reverse may be true.

Often the term attention is used interchangeably with other terms such as alertness, vigilance, or effort. This creates confusion and does not assist the therapist in identifying deficits and designing treatment programs. These and other related terms therefore are defined in an effort to clarify related concepts, as follows:

Alerting. More related to the periphery, preparing the individual to mobilize to attention, and theoretically functions through different neurological systems from attention;[14] a fluctuating condition of the central nervous system.[12]

Attention. Means by which one can orient in order to receive incoming information;[7] contains the three components of alertness, selectivity and effort. Subcategories of attention include the following:[7]

- Focused attention. The ability to respond to different kinds of stimulation; it involves direction and orientation
- Sustained attention. Vigilance; maintaining attention for a long time
- Selective attention. Activating and inhibiting responses selectively; involves discrimination of stimulus information and differentiating responses
- Alternating attention. (attentional flexibility). Alternating back and forth between mental tasks, ex. chopping vegetables while periodically checking food on the stove[15]
- Divided attention. Ability to do several things at once
- Concentration. The ability to do mental work while attending, the process of active encoding in working memory.[7]

- Divided attention deficit. Occurs "when controlled processing is in use and where the limitations of the system fail to accommodate all the information necessary for optimal task performance."[12] This often results in patients becoming slow in processing and behavior and "overloaded" when they have to deal with several alternatives.
- Focused attention deficit. Occurs "when an automatic response is replaced by a controlled response,"[12] eg, walking after a C.V.A.
- Selective attention. The process of choosing some items of information rather than others; some items affect awareness, memory, and behavior more than nonselected items that may be present at the same time.[12]
- Vigilance. The ability to sustain attention over a period of time.[7] Thirty seconds is considered a vigilant period in a mental status examination;[16] a control process that coordinates functional components of attention (alertness, arousal, and selectivity) to direct attention to significant features of the environment. **Note**: It is this aspect of attention that appears particularly vulnerable to brain damage.[17]

Attentional deficits have been linked to the reticular activating system, frontal and temporal lobes and the limbic system.[16,18-21] Traumatic brain-injured patients often exhibit poor concentration and divided attention as well as a general "mental slowing."[9,17,22] C.V.A. and T.B.I. patients often complain that they cannot continue what they have started and cannot focus on a problem or situation. The individual "...drifts further away before anything significant is accomplished.[17]

Any type of attentional deficit common to the C.V.A. or T.B.I. patient will impair learning and all aspects of daily functioning.[15,23] Because memory, problem solving and other higher intellectual functions all have an attentional component, attention should always be evaluated at the beginning of a functional cognitive evaluation.

Evaluation of Attention

TEST 1: TEST OF EVERYDAY ATTENTION (T.E.A.)[24]*

Description:
There are eight subtests of the T.E.A.: map search, elevator counting, elevator counting with distractions, visual elevator, elevator counting with reversal, telephone search, telephone search while counting, and lottery.

Clinical strengths[24]
1. The T.E.A. gives a broad-based measure of the most important clinical and theoretical aspects of attention; no other existing test of attention does this.
2. The T.E.A. has three versions which allow testing on three successive occasions with parallel material.
3. The T.E.A. can be used analytically to identify different patterns of attentional breakdown.
4. The T.E.A. has a very wide range of application, ranging from patients with early Alzheimer's disease to young normal subjects.
5. It is the only test of attention based largely on everyday materials; the real-life scenario means that most patients enjoy the test and find it relevant to their problems of adjustment in everyday life.

---

*Reproduced with permission from Thames Valley Test Co., Burly St. Edmunds, England. Distributed by Northern Speech Services Inc., 117 N. Elm Street, PO Box 1247, Gaylord, MI 49735.

Table 8-1. Reliability[24]
Pearson Correlations

Subtest	Normal Controls (N=119): Version A with B	Normal Controls (N=39): Version B with C	Stroke Patients (N=74): Version A with B
Map Search (one minute)	0.83	8.87	0.84
Map Search (two minutes)	0.86	0.80	0.85
Elevator Counting	ceiling effect	ceiling effect	0.88
Elevator Counting with Distractions	0.71	0.68	0.83
Visual Elevator- raw accuracy score	0.71	0.76	0.90
Visual Elevator- timing score	0.79	0.70	not calculated
Elevator Counting with Reversal	0.66	0.68	not administered
Telephone Search- raw score	0.86	0.90	0.78
Telephone Search While Counting- dual task decrement	0.59	0.61	0.41 (see text)
Lottery	ceiling effect	ceiling effect	0.77

Reliability:
Test-retest reliability coefficients are given in Table 8-1 on versions A and B for 118 subjects from the normal sample and for 74 subjects of the C.V.A. sample. In addition, test-retest reliability figures are given for a subsample of the normal sample who were given version C a week after receiving version B.

Validity:
Extensive validity measures were generated with various populations and other existing tests which purported to measure attention. Details of these studies are contained in the test manual.[24]

Procedure:
Subtest 1 - Map search is provided as an example.*

---

*Reproduced with permission from Thames Valley Test Co., Burly St. Edmunds, England. Distributed by Northern Speech Services Inc., 117 N. Elm Street, PO Box 1247, Gaylord, MI 49735.

General introduction to the test:

Subjects are asked to imagine that they are on vacation (holiday) in the USA, in Philadelphia. They will carry out a number of everyday tasks during this imaginary vacation (holiday). Each task has its own scenario. The general verbatim instruction for the introduction to the test is as follows. The wording is to be followed verbatim, though the tester must judge when to re-emphasize an instruction that is unclear to the subject.

Say:

"We are interested in your concentration on a range of everyday tasks. I want you to imagine that you are on a long trip to Philadelphia (United States). I will ask you to do various tasks such as looking at maps and looking up telephone directories while you are on this imaginary trip. Let me explain the first task."

SUBTESTS

Map Search

This timed, visual search task involves searching a map for a total of two minutes and circling a particular symbol on the map when located. After 1 minute, subjects are given a different colored pen to enable the tester to count the number of targets located in 1 minute versus the total for 2 minutes.

The symbols are in the cuebook, according to which version of the test (A, B or C) is being given. There are two maps of the Philadelphia area. Each map has two types of symbols. There are eighty of each type of symbol. On each map, only one symbol is the target for a given version of the subtest. The cuebook is left open at the target symbol in front of the subject during the subtest, to remind him or her of the symbol being sought.

- For Version A, the fork and knife on Version A map.
- For Version B, the screwdriver with wrench (spanner) on Version B & C map.
- For Version C, the gas (petrol) pump on Version B & C map.

Instructions:

Say:

"The symbol here (show symbol from cuebook) shows where restaurants (or garages, or gas [petrol] stations) can be found in the Philadelphia area. There are many symbols like this on the map."

Point to one at left side of map. Also, indicate to subject that the symbols are found all over the map, left and right, top and bottom. Check that the subject can see the symbol clearly. Turn the map over so the subject cannot scan it while you give further instructions.

Say:

"Let's say you are with a family member or a friend. They are driving while you are navigating. You want to know where restaurants (or garages, or gas [petrol] stations) are located in case you decide to stop for a meal (or to get you car checked, or to fill up). What I would like you to do is to look at the map for two minutes and circle as many symbols as you can. I will stop you once when a minute has gone by to ask you to swap pens. OK?"

When the subject indicates that he has understood (reiterate the instructions if he has not) turn the map over to reveal the symbols, give him a red pen and begin timing. After 1 minute, ask the subject to change pens and hand him a blue pen. At the end of 2 minutes, ask the subject to stop.

If the subject feels that he has completed the task before the 2 minute time limit, or if he assumes that he has done so by reaching the right hand edge of the map, ask him to continue searching for any symbols which he might have missed until the end of the time limit.

Common errors made by subjects:

Subjects usually comprehend this task very easily. Occasionally, subjects talk during the task, thereby slowing their performance. In this case, the assessor should try not to respond or simply say "Remember to find as many as you can." In some instances, subjects stop searching after they have found only a few targets, apparently finding it difficult to persist. The assessor should make the same basic comment as above, perhaps with some encouragement: "You are doing fine so far. Keep finding as many as you can for a bit longer" or "There are quite a few symbols, can you find more?"

Scoring:
Slip the Version A, B or C template into the plastic folder over the map with the printed side up. Then count the number of target symbols circled in red. This is the 1 minute score. Then count the number circled in blue, and add this to the red total. This is the 2 minute score.

TEST 2: DYNAMIC INTERACTIONAL ASSESSMENT[13,25,26]

Description:
This is not a single test, but qualitative analysis of how the patient performs on a given task. Three components of the evaluation process are: awareness questioning strategy, investigation and task grading, and response to cuing.

Awareness questioning

General questions:
"Have you noticed any changes in your memory?"
"Have you noticed any changes in your attention?"
"How would you rate your ability to concentrate/remember compared to before the injury?" (100%, 75%, 50%, 25%, 0%)

Prediction/estimation questions:
"On a scale of 1 to 4, how difficult do you think this task will be?"
(1 = very difficult, 2 = difficult, 3 = easy, 4 = very easy)
"To what extent do you feel that your ability to perform this type of task has changed?"
(no change, slight change, definite change, big change)
"Out of 20 items, how many do you think you will remember?"
"Do you think you would have performed any differently before the injury?"

Strategy investigation
Observe how the individual performs a task and question the individual's responses without suggesting the answers. The patient's response to strategy questions will supplement clinical observations of performance and provide the therapist with information on the patient's thought process.

Task grading response to cuing
If the patient has trouble with 50% of the task, change one parameter.[13] Begin testing at mid level.

Procedures:
Toglia has applied her theoretical concepts to five different categories of attentional tasks. Table 8-2 is a sample of this application.

TEST 3: CLINICAL OBSERVATION AND ACTIVITY ANALYSIS

General guidelines for evaluation:
1. Identify the components of attention (eg, alerting, selectivity, effort) that are intact and those that are impaired.
2. Observe the patient in a number of settings and activities at different times during the day. Position change (lying, sitting) can also affect attention.
3. Establish functional baseline measures. Consider the frequency and severity of the problem. Select relevant functional tasks as the basis for the evaluation and reassessment.

Table 8-2. Attentional Flexibility Tasks[13]

Task Level	Sample Tasks	Response (Indicate # and letter)	Sample Cues
1. Follows one change	A. Copy the following: mmmmmmnnn	___ Follows changes in task smoothly	General feedback: *Are you sure you followed the sequence?*
	B. Add these pairs of numbers. Now subtract these numbers. 2 4 5 6 7 3 5 5 9 3 7 2	___ Occasionally (25%) errors observed following a change. ___ Occasionally (25%) errors observed following a change. ___ Errors observed following a change 50% of the time. ___ Errors observed following a change more than 50% of the time	Specific feedback: *Some of the sequence is correct but there are a few places where you (e.g. added instead of subtracted)* Self-initiated strategy:
	C. Playing cards spread face up all over the table: Turn over the even-numbered cards. Now turn over the odd-numbered cards.		
2. Alternates between two different sequences or responses	A. Copy the following: mmmmmmmmmm	Observed behaviors following change: ___ No change in behavior ___ Becomes distracted ___ Required redirection to task ___ Perseveration ___ Slowness, hesitation ___ Impulsive	*Can you think of a way to make it easier to follow changes?* Provide Strategy: *For example, this time try to say it aloud to help you* General feedback: *Are you sure you followed the sequence?*
	B. Add the first 2 pairs of numbers. Subtract the next 2 pairs of numbers and continue alternating. 2 4 7 3 6 7 9 2 12 4 11 6 13 5 15 3	___ Remains goal directed ___ Becomes distracted (1-2x, 3-4x, >5x) but unable to redirect self back to task ___ Occasional redirection needed ___ Frequent redirection needed ___ Continual redirection needed ___ Attention span is adequate ___ Attention span is inadequate (indicate high)	Specific feedback: *Some of the sequence is correct but there are a few places where you (e.g. added instead of subtracted)* Self-initiated strategy: *Can you think of a way to make it easier to follow changes?* Provide strategy: *For example, this time try to sat it aloud to help you.*
	C. Playing cards: Playing cards in rows, face up. Turn over the odd cards, but as soon as you get to a J, Q, or K card, switch to turning over even cards. When you get to the next J, Q, or K card, switch back to odd cards and so on.		

Table 8-2. Attentional Flexibility Tasks (continued)

Task Level	Sample Tasks	Response (Indicate # and letter)	Sample Cues

3. Generates alternate responses or ideas	A. If you had $9.85, tell me all the different lunches you could order.
	B. Tell me all the different coin combinations that will make $1.05.
	C. Playing cards: Tell me all the different card combinations that add up to 21.
		____ Fluctuations in performance
		____ Performance deteriorates at end of task
		____ Response speed modulated
		____ Perseverative
		____ Impulsive
		____ Slow
			Sample task modifications:
			   Change task level
			   Increase saliency of cue for "change"
			   Decrease frequency of changes
			   Decrease number of stimuli
			   Eliminate time limit
			   Decrease selection demands

Adapted from Toglia, J.P. (1992b). Cognitive rehabilitation: A dynamic instructional approach. Supplement manual to workshop conducted at New York Hospital - Cornell Medical Center, New York. Reproduced with permission from Toglia J.P., Mercy College, Occupational Therapy Program, 555 Broadway, Dobbs Ferry, New York 10522.

Specific areas or questions to consider and evaluate:
1. Which sensory systems are affected? Visual? Auditory?
2. What are the duration and frequency of the patient's attentional abilities?
3. Under what environmental conditions can the patient attend to a task? When does attention begin to break down?
4. What are some behavioral indications of the patient's inattention?
5. Does the patient have memory problems? Does he have problem solving difficulties? Decreased processing? Are these or related problems caused in part by decreased attention?
6. Are there any tasks or areas that seem to particularly interest the patient and therefore increase his attention?
7. Is processing occurring only at a conscious level as opposed to a normal combination of automatic and conscious?

Scoring:
Nonstandardized. The foregoing and similar questions can be incorporated into a checklist or used in conjunction with a frequency rating scale (eg, always/sometimes/rarely/never). To improve validity, rule out auditory and language problems as the causes of poor performance.

Treatment for Attention Deficits

Utilizing a Remedial Approach:

1. Identify which type or types of attention are affected and target these areas in treatment.[9]
2. Provide cues that help the patient access and use previous knowledge to organize new information.[13] This can enhance attention.
3. Provide a behavioral frame of reference to attention training.[27] For example, the patient receives a token when he or she maintains attention for a pre-determined time. A certain amount of tokens are exchanged for a previously agreed upon reward.
4. Motivation and the patient's emotional state can alter his or her ability to attend and remember.[13] It is important, therefore, to provide training which is motivating to the patient.[28]
5. Apply concepts from the dynamic interactional frame of reference and alter the task and/or environment to change the patient's level of attention.[13] Identify what task level and type of environment causes decreased attention. Start activities at this stage and progress. Tasks emphasizing the different aspects of attention can each be graded from simple to complex.[13]
6. Provide training to help the patient develop active listening skills by:[29]
   a. maintaining eye contact
   b. as much as possible, maintain a body posture that is erect but relaxed, which indicates interest and attention
7. In an attempt to utilize sensory input (visual, tactile, auditory) in relation to motor output (eg, attention to task, participation in task), provide controlled sensory cuing with the patient, subsequently demonstrating active interaction with the environment. Initially provide sensory cuing separately, eg, visual, auditory or tactile. Once the patient is able to respond to single system cues, provide multisystem cues.[30]
8. Utilize computer software which has been specifically designed for the remediation of attention deficits.[9,27,31]

9. Review with the physician what medication the patient is taking. Discuss what medication can help or hurt attention skills.[32] Research has shown that medication can be used to improve patient attention.[33]
10. Provide table top graded activities which focus on attentional skills (ie, cancellation tasks, mazes).
11. Teach the patient to actively scan his environment, seek out the presence of cues and identify them.[34,35]

Utilizing an Adaptive Approach:

1. Many theorists believe that the "…regulation of attention is largely dependent on subvocal or inner speech."[36] Verbal mediation by the patient to compensate for attention deficit has been found to be an effective compensation strategy.[37,38]
   a. The patient can be taught statements to prepare himself to listen and ask for repetition if his attention strays[39] (eg, "I must really concentrate and look at the person speaking to me").
   b. Have the patient vocalize step by step as he performs a task. Progress to subvocalization (patient silently vocalizes), thereby internalizing the technique.[39]
2. If necessary, staff and family should speak slowly and in short sentences with pauses to allow time for processing.[32] Ask the patient to paraphrase what he or she has just heard and repeat information if needed. Teach the patient to cue others to speak more slowly and request repetition.
3. Adapt both the external and internal patient environment by reducing distracters.
   a. external — remove clutter, reduce noise level
   b. internal — reduce hunger, pain, anger, fatigue, etc. For example, adjust room temperature, provide rest periods. Teach the patient to shelve emotional internal distracters through techniques such as visual imagery.[29]
4. Adapt tasks in a way that information processing elements of a task are emphasized or highlighted.[40,41] For example, underline an important part of written directions, or make important elements visually bigger or a different color. This will help the patient discriminate different components of the learning task.[41]

Memory

Memory is not a simple function, but one that relates to learning and how we perceive our world. Whenever we try to remember something we are involving many other cognitive skills.[2] An individual's mood or level of motivation will also affect his memory function and the quality of new learning.[7] Memory may be impaired as a result of an attentional disorder, as one must be able to attend to and perceive something before it can be remembered.[17] Memory is essentially perception that has been stored at an earlier time and can then be brought forward. Memory loss can be general or relate to specific types of coded information, and any sense or combination of senses can elicit a recollection.[7,17,42,43]

No matter what definition one utilizes for memory, the underlying concept that it includes permanent change in the central nervous system, which can later be reproduced, appears to be universally accepted.[19] The constant interaction between an individual and the environment elicits memories, which can be retrieved in an exact or equivalent form.[19] Memory requires input from the environment (both internal and external), change within the central nervous system, maintenance of that change, and an output (behavioral or information) that somehow consistently relates to the input.[19]

The memory process begins with the input of sensations. The individual selectively attends to the environment depending on his interests at the time of a given sensory input from the environment. This process of sensory memory, which is the first phase of an individual's information processing, has the capability to process enormous amounts of information for brief duration.[7] Sensory memory is generally broken down into iconic or sensory visions and echoic or auditory sensory memory.[7] If information is distorted at this first stage of processing, then the encoding process in all other areas of memory will be adversely affected.[7]

The process continues from sensory memory to *working memory*, where information is retained by mental repetition. This process is termed *rehearsal*. Working memory can deal with approximately seven pieces of information at a time, and is considered part of a control mechanism for higher intellectual processing and functions.[7,17,44,45] From working memory, items are encoded and consolidated into long-term memory. Encoding begins with selective attention and is the means by which information is transformed in working memory so that it can be stored efficiently in long-term memory.[7] Consolidation is "...the integration of new memories within the individual's existing cognitive linguistic schema or framework."[2] The consolidation process can take minutes or hours and can be stored in long-term memory—in some cases for life.[19,20,44] The deeper working memory processes information, the better it is remembered.[7]

Retrieval of stored information is the final aspect of the memory process. There are two stages of retrieval: 1) the search for available information, and 2) the directing of an appropriate verbal or motor response.[7] Iconic retrieval is accomplished through a simple read out, whereas working memory retrieval is dependent on rehearsal ability.[7] Working memory for purely visual tasks depends on the ability to sustain a visual image and scan it.[7]

Various types of memory play an important role in an individual's ability to function and communicate successfully.[11] The patient with a C.V.A or T.B.I. can have any aspect of impaired memory. T.B.I. patients, for example, often lose the ability to automatically rehearse and encode information.[7] This inability in turn affects future abstraction and/or the ability to learn from one's errors.[7] C.V.A. or T.B.I. patients also often have difficulty with "meta-memory," or the ability to "remember to remember."[10] These patients have difficulty cuing themselves.

Evaluation of Memory

TEST 1: RIVERMEAD BEHAVIORAL MEMORY TEST (RBMT)[46]*

Description:
Test of everyday memory functioning. Test items involve either remembering to carry out

Table 8-3. Standardized Profile Scoring for the RBMT[46]
(Raw scores are indicated in the body of the table.)

Standardized Profile Score

Item		2 points	1 point	0 points
1 & 2	First and	4	3	0-2
	Second Name	4	3	0-2
3	Belonging	4	3	0-2
4	Appointment	2	1	0
5	Pictures	10	9	0-8
6a	Story (immediate)	6 or more	4-5.5	3.5 or less
6b	Story (delayed)	4 or more	2-3.5	1.5 or less
7	Faces	5	4	0-3
8a	Route (immediate)	5	4	0-3
8b	Route (delayed)	5	4	0-3
9	Message	6	5	0-4
10	Orientation	9	8	0-7
11	Date	1	1 day out	2 or more days out

some everyday task, or retaining the type of information needed for adequate everyday functioning. There are four parallel versions of the test, which negates any practice effect due to repeated testing. Items are presented in sequence so that early items can be recalled by the patient later in testing.

Scoring:
There are two scoring systems for the RBMT: Screening Score and Standardized Profile Score. For the Screening score, each item is scored pass (1) or fail (0), with a total possible score of 12. Rating is then made as follows:
10, 11, 12 - Normal
7, 8, 9 - Poor memory
3, 4, 5, 6 - moderately impaired memory
0, 1, 2 - severely impaired
The Standardized Profile Score is computed from the raw score as indicated in Table 8-3.

Reliability:
Inter-rater reliability was established with 40 subjects and two raters with 100% agreement between both raters. Parallel-form reliability was established by giving two versions of the test to 118 patients. The correlation between the two scores was .78 for the screening score and .85 for the profile score.

Validity:
1) The test was given to brain-damaged patients and controls, with the patients having substantially lower scores than the control subjects. 2) Performance on the RBMT was corre-

Table 8-4. Correlation Matrix;
Memory Test Scores for Patients[46]

	Screen	Profile	R.M.W.	R.M.F.	Digits Forward	Digits Backward	P.A.L.T.	Corsi	Sem Proc Correct	Sem Proc. Att.
Screening Total	-	0.97 ***	0.60 ***	0.41 ***	0.29 ***	0.24 ***	0.60 ***	0.28 **	0.24 **	0.22 **
Profile Total		-	0.63 ***	0.43 ***	0.30 ***	0.27 ***	0.62 ***	0.28 ***	0.22 ***	0.20 **
Recognition Memory for Words (RMW)			-	0.37 ***	0.29 ***	0.31 ***	0.48 ***	0.19 *	0.16 *	0.13 NS
Recognition Memory for Faces (RMF)				-	0.17 *	0.14 N.S.	0.22 **	0.27 ***	0.19 *	0.19 *
Digits Forward					-	0.56 ***	0.42 ***	0.21 **	0.27 ***	0.31 ***
Digits Backward						-	0.44 ***	0.41 ***	0.26 ***	0.26 ***
Paired Associate Learning Test (PALT)							-	0.17 *	0.23 **	0.24 **
Corsi Blocks								-	0.22 **	0.21 **
Semantic Processing Correct									-	0.97 ***
Semantic Processing Attempted										-

***p < .001; **p < .01; *p < .05; N.S. Not Significant

Reproduced with permission from Thames Valley Test Co., Burly St. Edmunds, England. Distributed by Speech Services Inc., 117 Elm St., P.O. Box 1247, Gaylord, Michigan 48735.

lated with performance on a number of standard memory tests. Table 8-4 shows the inter-correlations between performance on the various tests. Additional areas were examined, such as sex differences, intelligence, age etiology, aphasia, and perceptual problems. Detailed results of these studies are contained in the test manual supplements 2 & 3.[46]

Procedure:
The following are examples of test items of version A of the RBMT.*

Items 1 & 2: First and Second Name*
The subject is shown a photographic portrait and asked to remember the first and second name of the person in the photograph. Say:
"What I want you to do is to remember this person's name (show photograph). Her name is Catherine Taylor. Can you repeat the name? Later on I am going to ask you what her name is."
The photograph is then placed face downwards on the table.

Item 3: Appointment*
The alarm is set for 20 minutes and the subject is required to ask a particular question relating to the near future, when the alarm sounds. Say:
"I am going to set this alarm to go off in 20 minutes." (Demonstrate alarm and set.) "When it rings, I want you to ask me about your next appointment. Say something like, 'Can you tell me when I have to to see you again?', or words to that effect."

TEST 2: CONTEXTUAL MEMORY TEST (CMT)[47]

Description:
The CMT is intended as a supplement to other measures of memory and cognition. It is designed to objectively measure awareness and strategy use in adults with memory impairment and/or screen patients for memory impairment which may require further testing. Test items are functionally oriented. Areas covered are:
1. Awareness of memory capacity (through general questioning, prediction of memory capacity prior to task performance, and estimation of memory capacity following task performance.
2. Recall of line drawn objects (immediate and delayed).
3. Strategy use, ie, the ability to describe use of strategies and the ability to benefit from a strategy provided by the examiner.

Scoring:
There are three recall raw scores—immediate, delayed and total recall—which are converted to standard scores. Prediction scores are generated through comparison with the actual recall score. The estimation score is also calculated through comparison with the actual recall score. Strategy use is examined through the effect of context, the total strategy use, and the order of recall.

Reliability:
Parallel form reliability was conducted with the two forms of the test, with reliability estimates ranging from 0.73 to 0.81. Quasi (partial) test-retest reliability ranged from 0.74 to 0.87 for the control group and from 0.85 to 0.94 for the group with brain injury. The Rasch method was utilized to generate additional reliability measures, which are covered in the test manual. Parallel form reliability for prediction and strategy scores was also generated and described in the test manual.

Validity:
Concurrent validity was determined by examining the correlation between the CMT and Rivermead Behavioral Memory Test. Correlations ranged from 0.80 to 0.84. The Rasch analysis was used to chart the individual abilities and item difficulties of the controls and brain injury subjects. Results are described in the test manual.

---

*Reproduced with permission from Thames Valley Test Co., Burly St. Edmunds, England. Distributed by Northern Speech Services Inc., 117 N. Elm Street, PO Box 1247, Gaylord, MI 49735.

Author's note: Toglia has also provided in the test manual a section for interpreting test results (Patterns of Performance) and applying these results to treatment.

TEST 3: AUTOBIOGRAPHICAL MEMORY INTERVIEW (A.M.I.)[48]*

Description:
This test provides an assessment of patient's personal remote memory, including identifying the pattern of any deficit and its temporal gradient. Test items require the patient to recall facts from his past life, relating to childhood, early adult life, and more recent facts. Each subtest is scored out of 21 points.

Procedure:
The following items are examples from each section of the overall test battery.

Section A: Childhood (Period Before School)

Personal semantic questions:
1. Ask the subject for the address where he or she was living before going to school.
2 points for the full address
1 point for the street and town only
1/2 point for the town or street only

2. Ask the subject the names of three friends or neighbors from the period before the subject went to school.
1 point for each surname
1/2 point each if first name only

Section B: Early Adult Life

Personal semantic questions:
3. Ask the subject for the name of his or her main secondary (or high) school. If the subject attended several secondary (or high) schools, ask which one was attended when the subject was 13 years old.
1 point for the correct name
Note: If the subject only attended one school, it can be scored twice if correct, but separate incidents must be given for primary and secondary schools with a total of six names of friends or teachers.

Section C: Recent life (Present Hospital or Institution)

Personal or semantic questions:
Note: It is expected that most subjects will be seen in a hospital or institution (eg, a research institute). However, if the subject is being seen in another location (eg, own home) the questions should be rephrased to accomodate this.
4. Ask the subject for the name of the hospital or place (eg, institution) where he or she is currently being seen.
1 point for the correct name of the hospital or institution.

Scoring:
Scoring is computed by a "cut off" which is related to the number of standard deviations from the norm. Cut off scores are described in Table 8-5.

---

*Reproduced with permission from Thames Valley Test Co., Burly St. Edmunds, England. Distributed by Northern Speech Services Inc., 117 N. Elm Street, PO Box 1247, Gaylord, MI 49735.

Table 8-5. Cut-off Scores[46]

	Personal semantic schedule				Autobiographical incidents schedule			
	Childhood	Young adult	Recent	Total	Childhood	Young adult	Recent	Total
Acceptable range	16-21	17-21	19-21	54-63	6-9	7-9	7-9	19-27
Borderline	14-15	16	18	50-52	5	5-6	6	16-18
Probably abnormal	12-13	15	-	48-49	4	4	-	13-15
Definitely abnormal	≤11	≤14	≤17	≤47	≤3	≤3	≤5	≤12

Reliability:
Inter-rater reliability was established with three raters with correlation's between .83 and .86.

Validity:
1. Examined how well the test discriminated between amnesic patients and healthy controls.
2. Examined the intercorrelation between different remote memory tasks in the total patient group.
3. Compared the pattern of temporal gradients across different tests of remote memory.
4. Checked the authenticity of the memories produced.

TEST 4: THE SUBJECTIVE MEMORY QUESTIONNAIRE[49]

Description:
This scale consists of 43 items relating to everyday life. These items cover areas such as people's names, facts about people, film titles, jokes, and directions to get somewhere.

Scoring:
Two different 5-point rating scales are utilized. The first 36 items are answered on a "very good" to "very bad" scale. Items 37 to 43 are temporal and are answered on a "very rarely" to "very often" scale.
To improve validity, rule out attentional and language related problems as causes of poor performance.

Reliability:
Test-retest reliability has been established (p<0.001) on this questionaire.[49] Item correlation also indicated "high positive item to test correlations."[49]

TEST 5: CLINICAL OBSERVATION AND ACTIVITY ANALYSIS

General guidelines for evaluation:
1. Identify the aspects of memory that are impaired and those that are relatively intact.
2. Observe the patient in a number of settings.
3. Consider the amount of structure versus nonstructure within the environment.
4. Consider the time interval between stimulus and recall (ie, immediate, short-term, and long-term).

5. Establish functional baseline measures. Consider the frequency and severity of the problem as it relates to function. Select relevant functional areas or tasks as the basis for evaluation and reassessment.

Specific areas and questions to consider and evaluate:

1. Which sensory system is affected? For instance, immediate recall can be tested for different sensory systems as follows:[42,50,51]
    a. Visual. The patient is asked to reproduce simple geometric figures, which are presented for 5 to 10 seconds and then covered.[42,50,51] **Note**: if a person's perceptual abilities are impaired, it is likely that this will affect memory for visual material and the ability to use visually based strategies to assist in memory problems.[52]
    b. Kinesthetic. The patient is asked to reproduce a series of hand positions presented to him.[42]
    c. Auditory. The patient is asked to reproduce a series of rhythmic taps.[42] **Note**: if the patient is aphasic, verbal memory and the ability to use verbal memory strategies are likely to be affected.
2. Is nonverbal memory impaired? Verbal memory?
3. Is memory loss global or modality specific?
4. Is it a learning or a performance problem? Can the patient improve with practice?
5. Can the patient utilize identified strategies for improved memory?
6. Is it a problem of learning new information or recalling old information?
7. Is the patient aware of his memory problem?
8. Which memory processes are affected? Does the patient have trouble identifying as well as reproducing (recall versus recognition)?
9. Is it a semantic memory loss? Is it episodic?
10. Does the patient have difficulty with free recall?
11. Does the patient have difficulty with serial learning (ie, remembering sequences)?
12. Does the patient have difficulty with paired associates (ie, remembering relationships)?

Scoring:

Nonstandardized. The foregoing or similar questions can be incorporated into a checklist (yes/no) or used in conjunction with a frequency rating scale (eg, always/sometimes/rarely/never). These questions or checklists should be used in a variety of environments and tasks. Comparisons of performance can then be made. This information can then be incorporated into the treatment plan.

To improve validity, rule out perceptual, language, and attentional deficits as causes of poor performance.

Treatment for Memory Deficits

Utilizing a Remedial Approach:

The following general treatment principles should be applied in the remedial approach to memory deficits:

1. The remediation of short-term memory will have limited effect in early stages of recovery.[7] Attentional processes and sensory memory should be addressed first.
2. Attention training results in improved memory in many patients.[9]

3. Along with attention and concentration, rehearsal is a necessary antecedent of memory retraining.[7]

attention	$\rightarrow$	rehearsal
$\downarrow$		$\downarrow$
can select information to rehearse		maintains information to encode and store it in long-term memory

4. The patient must relearn rehearsal skills before any other form of working memory training can work. The therapist must evaluate how many rehearsals are required to bring the patient's memory to average levels.
5. Teach the patient to rehearse information in a manner that will ensure that it transfers to long-term memory so that it can be retrieved at a later time.[7]
6. Effective encoding of information is required for future recall.[9] If the material is well analyzed, recall at a later time will be easier.
7. Identify and characterize patient's preserved memory abilities and build memory retraining strategies around them.[53]
8. Research has shown that it is possible to teach a patient with severe memory loss different kinds of domain specific learning that can be applied to A.D.L.[54,55] This is only accomplished if the procedure is consistent, the job is broken down into component steps and the patient is taught each component directly.
9. Organization facilitates recall.[7] The C.V.A. or T.B.I. patient may lose the ability to organize automatically (refer to section on organization and planning).
10. Straight repetitive drills do not appear to generalize to untrained memory or functional memory outside the clinic.[2,56] Repetition with the use of vanishing cues, however, has been shown to be effective.[55] Computer software with vanishing cues built into the program are especially helpful.
11. Utilize an indirect, direct or domain specific approach depending on the patient's awareness of memory loss, strategy use and recall status.[47] Please refer to references 25 and 47 for detailed information of the application of these concepts.

Utilizing an Adaptive Approach:

Assist the patient in developing and effectively utilizing both internal and external memory aids and strategies to compensate for memory loss. The following are examples of strategies and external aids which can be utilized:[2,7,13,19,28,29,39,43,44,46,47,52,55,57-72]

Memory Strategies:

active listening— Refer to the section on Treatment of Attention Deficits
note taking—Lists, schedules, instructions directions

audio taping—This technique is especially useful with patients with poor motor skills, slow information processing and decreased vision.

rehearsal— The more sensory systems which are used, the more likely the information will be remembered. Use methods which are the patient's best methods of encoding. This method is only effective when used in combination with other strategies.

association—Two new pieces of information can be associated or new information can be associated with old information. Associations can be gained from all sensory modalities. An emotional association can also assist in recall.

pegging— This technique can be used to assist the patient in remembering someone or to assist him in remembering various tasks. For example:

S - shopping

L - laundry

E - eat lunch

E - exercise

P - pick up children at school

To remember someone, pick out a key feature to associate with that person and attach a name or object to it. For example, overweight → barrel → Darryl.

rhyming mnemonics— A word that rhymes with the word or information to be recalled is utilized, eg, fun-sun, heaven-seven.

P.Q.R.S.T. Method[64]

Preview—The patient skims the material to learn the general content.

Question—The patient asks himself key questions about the content.

Read—The patient reads the information with the goal of answering the question.

State—The patient repeats or rehearses the information read.

Test—The patient tests himself by answering the questions he posed previously.

loci— The patient forms associations between locations and the information to be remembered. The patient takes an imaginary walk around his or her favorite room and envisions items to be recalled in various locations, ie, bread on the table, milk on the T.V., etc.

chunking and grouping — This is a way to organize information to be recalled. For example: categories (grouping meat products in a grocery list), object properties (color, size, shape), function (knives in a drawer), origins (items that grow on trees).

mental retracing— Some research has indicated this is the most frequently utilized internal memory strategy by patients.[73]

visual imagery — Patients with left hemisphere brain damage may find this to be an effective tool.[7]

story method — The patient forms a story about the words or phrases he is to remember.[45]

self-reference— The patient judges how the material relates to him. This has been found to assist retention more than relating it to others.[43]

External Aids

General principles of effective external cuing include the following:
1. Give the cuing as close as possible to the time the action is required.
2. Make it active.
3. Be specific about what is required.
4. Retrieval cues that are similar to the ones used in the original learning process can be especially helpful to recall.
5. Questioning the patient during presentation appears to assist in retention.
6. If using a device:
   a. Make it portable. The device should be able to store as many cues as possible.
   b. It should have as wide a time range as possible.
   c. It should be easy to use and not be dependent on any other instrument.
   d. Training for the use of an external memory device should include:[71]
      - acquisition — how to use the device
      - application — when and where to use the device
      - adaptation — learning to use the device in novel situation

Specific external devices include:
1. storage devices — diaries, notebooks*, lists, calculators and computers
2. cuing devices — alarm clocks, bell timers, watch alarms
3. structured environments — labeled drawers, cabinets, or doors

Harrel et al[29] offer an eight-step treatment model for the application of strategies and aids as well as memory retraining tasks as follows:
1. Select a task or strategy.
   a. choose one for which the patient can experience success
   b. follow a hierarchy of skills, ie, attention and concentration before recall of information
   c. make the task relevant to the patient's life (ie, age, interest, etc.)
   d. make tasks measurable (ie, time to complete, percentage or number completed, number of strategies used, etc.)
2. Measure the patient's performance without any assistance given.
3. Set relevant goals, with the patient if possible. Identify both short and long term goals.
4. Choose and teach a strategy or way to approach the task. Use a strategy that is most applicable to the patient's real world.

---

*Note: Research has shown that patients are more likely to use a memory notebook if it is easily distinguishable from other folders and notebooks, for example, bright orange or red.

5. Provide the patient with opportunities to practice new learning on a regular basis until the strategy is overlearned.

6. When the patient has mastered the strategy, or plateaued, decide if the goal has been reached or needs to be altered.

7. Practice transfer and generalization in a hierarchical manner as follows:
   a. transfer to a different task in therapy
   b. transfer to the next therapy session
   c. transfer to a different type of therapy or situation
   d. generalize to the real world

8. Practice the strategy in different settings, especially real world settings.

The following is an example of how to apply this model to a specific recall task:[29]

Task: Immediate recall of short articles.[29]

Description: The client and therapist choose a short article to read. Each presentation increases in length (eg, from 2 to 20 paragraphs), each article being exposed for the same length of time (eg, 3 to 5 minutes). After presentation, the client can respond by writing, pointing, or reciting orally. Materials: Therapists can use articles from magazines, newspapers, short stories, books, essays, poems, and so forth.

Scoring: Percentage of information remembered from the article.

Baseline: Highest percentage of material recalled from the article.

Strategies: Chunking, highlighting, note taking, outlining, reading aloud (and audiotaping for repetition).

Example: Short newspaper or magazine article.

Variations:
- Types of articles can be varied from concrete to abstract, from old information that the client already knows to entirely new information, and so forth.
- Can be used as a recognition task by giving the client multiple-choice questions to answer at the end; the client can also recall information independent of cues.
- The task can be used for delayed recall by asking the client to remember information several minutes, days, or weeks later.
- Scoring can be done with the highest percentage of information recalled.

Generalizations: Manuals (car, appliances, computer), speeches, materials for class or work.

References

1. Rabbit P. Changes in problem solving ability in old age. In: Birren J, Schaie K (eds.). *Handbook of Psychology of Aging.* New York, Van Nostrand Reinhold Co.; 1977.
2. Sohlberg MM, Mateer CA. *Introduction To Cognitive Rehabilitation: Theory and Practice.* New York, The Guilford Press; 1989.
3. Deitz J, Tovar VS, Beeman C, Thorn DW, Trevisan MS. The test of orientation for rehabilitation patients: Test-retest reliability. *The Occupational Journal of Research.* 1992;12(3):173-185.
4. High WM, Levin HS, Gary HE. Recovery of orientation following closed head injury. *J of Clin and Experimental Neuropsychology.* 1990;12(5):703-714.
5. Itzkovich M, Arerback S, Belazar. *Lowenstein Occupational Therapy Cognitive Assessment.* Pequanock, NJ, Maddack Inc.
6. McNeny R, Dise J. Reality orientation therapy. In: Rosenthal M, Griffith ER, Bond MR, Miller JD (eds.). *Rehabilitation of the Adult with Traumatic Brain Injury.* Philadelphia, FA Davis Co.; 1983.
7. Parente R, Anderson J. *Retraining Memory: Techniques and Applications.* Houston, CSY Publishing; 1991.
8. Christiansen C. Occupational therapy: Intervention for life performance. In: Christiansen C, Baum C (eds). *Occupational Therapy: Overcoming Human Performance Deficits.* Thorofare, New Jersey, SLACK Inc.; 1991.
9. Sohlberg M, Mateer CA. Effectiveness of an attention-training program. *J Clinical Exper Neuropsych.* 1987;9(2):117-130.
10. Uomoto JM. Neuropsychological assessment and rehabilitation after brain injury. In: Craft GH, Berrol S (eds.). *Physical Medicine and Rehabilitation Clinics of North America.* Philadelphia, WB Saunders; 1992.
11. Adamovich BLB. Cognition, language, attention and information processing following closed head injury. In: Kreutzer JS, Wehman PH (eds.) *Cognitive Rehabilitation For Persons with Traumatic Brain Injury: A Functional Approach.* Baltimore, Paul H. Brooks Publishing Co.; 1991.
12. Wood RL. Management of attention disorders following brain injury. In: Wilson BA, Moffat N (eds.). *Clinical Management of Memory Problems.* Rockville, Maryland, Aspen Publishers; 1984.
13. Toglia JP. *Attention and Memory.* AOTA Self Study Series: Cognitive Rehabilitation. The American Occupational Therapy Association; 1994.
14. Breines E. *Perception: Its Development and Recapitulation.* Princeton, Geri-Rehab; 1981.
15. Okkema K. *Cognition and Perception in the Stroke Patient.* Gaithersburg, Aspen Publishers; 1993.
16. Strub RL, Black RW. *The Mental Status Examination in Neurology.* Philadelphia, FA Davis Co.; 1977.
17. Parker RS. *Traumatic Brain Injury and Neuropsychological Impairment.* New York, Springer-Verlag; 1990.
18. Ayres AJ. *Sensory Integration and Learning Disorders.* Los Angeles, Western Psychological Services; 1980.
19. Filskov S, Boll T. *Handbook of Clinical Neuropsychology.* New York, John Wiley & Sons, Inc.; 1981.
20. Luria AR. *Higher Cortical Functions in Man* (2nd edition). New York, Basic Books, Inc.; 1980.
21. Massey EW, Coffey CE. Frontal lobe personality syndromes: Ominous sequelae of head trauma. *Posrad Med.* 1983;73(5):99-106.
22. Grey JM. The remediation of attentional disorders following brain injury of acute onset. In: Wood RL, Fussey I (eds). *Cognitive Rehabilitation in Perspective.* London, Taylor & Frances; 1990.
23. Duchek J. Cognitive dimensions of performance. In: Christiansen C, Baum C (eds). *Occupational Therapy: Overcoming Human Performance Deficits.* Thorofare, New Jersey, SLACK Inc.; 1991.
24. Robertson I, Ward T, Ridgeway Y, Nimmo-Smith I. *The Test of Everyday Attention.* Bury St. Edwards, Thames Valley Test Co.; 1994.
25. Toglia JP. A dynamic interactional approach to cognitive rehabilitation. In: Katz N (ed.). *Cognitive Rehabilitation: Models For Intervention in Occupational Therapy.* Boston, Andover Med Pub.; 1992.
26. Toglia JP. Approaches to cognitive assessment of the brain-injured adult: Traditional methods and dynamic investigation. *Occup Ther Pract.* 1989;1(1):36-57.

27. Wood RL, Fussey I. *Cognitive Rehabilitation in Perspective.* London, Taylor and Francis; 1990.

28. Crovitz HF, Harvey MT, Horn RW. Problems in the acquisition of imagery mnemonics: Three brain-damaged cases. *Cortex.* 1979:225-234.

29. Harrell M, Parente F, Bellingrath EG, Lisicia KA. *Cognitive Rehabilitation of Memory.* Gaithersburg, MD, Aspen Publishers; 1992.

30. Diller L, Weinberg J. Differential aspects of attention in brain-damaged persons. *Percept Motor Skills.* 1972;35:71-81.

31. Skilleck C. Computer assistance in the management of memory and cognitive impairment. In: Wilson BA, Moffat N (eds.). *Clinical Management of Memory Problems.* Rockville, MD, Aspen Publishers; 1984.

32. Cohen RF, Mapou RL. Neuropsychological assessment for treatment planning: A hypothesis-testing approach. *J of Head Trauma Rehabil.* March 1988;3(1):12-23.

33. Tankle RS. Application of neuropsychological test results to interdisciplinary cognitive rehabilitation with head-injured adults. *J Head Trauma Rehabil.* 1988.3(1):24-32.

34. Piasetsky E, Ben-Yishay Y, Weinberg J. The systematic remediation of specific disorders: Selected application of methods derived in a clinical research setting. In: Trexler LE (ed.). *Cognitive Rehabilitation Conceptualization and Intervention.* New York, Plenum Press; 1982.

35. Rahmani L. The intellectual rehabilitation of brain-damaged patients. *Clin Neuropsychol.* 1982;4:44-45.

36. VanZomeren AH, Fasotti L. Impairments of attention in brain-damaged patients. In: VonSteinbuchel N, VonCramon DY and Poppel (eds.). *Neuropsychological Rehabilitation.* Berlin, Springer-Verlag; 1992.

37. McGlynn SM. Behavioral approaches to neuropsychological rehabilitation. *Psychological Bulletin.* 1990;108(3):420-4410.

38. Parente R. Executive Skills Training. In: *Retraining Cognition: Techniques and Application.* Parente R, Herrmann D (eds.) Gaithersburg, MD, Aspen Publications. (scheduled for publication 1996).

39. Webser J, Scott R. The effects of self-instructional training on attentional deficits following head injury. *Clin Neuropsychol.* 1983;5:69-74.

40. Dougherty PM, Radomski MV. *A Dynamic Assessment Approach for Adults with Brain Injury: The Cognitive Rehabilitation Workbook.* Gaithersburg, MD, Aspen Publishers; 1993.

41. Wood RL. Attention disorders in brain injury rehabilitation. *J Learning Disabilities.* June/July 1988;21(6):327-332.

42. Christenson AL. *Luria's Neuropsychological Investigation.* New York, Spectrum Publications; 1975.

43. Labowie-Vief, Gonda J. Cognitive strategy training and intellectual performance in the elderly. *J Gerontol.* 1967;31(3):327-332.

44. Baddeley AD. Memory theory and memory therapy. In: Wilson BA, Moffat N (eds.) *Clinical Management of Memory Problems.* Gaithersburg, MD, Aspen Publishers; 1984.

45. Gathsercole SE, Baddeley AD. *Working Memory and Language.* New Jersey, Lawrence Erlbaum Assoc.; 1993.

46. Wilson B, Cockburn J, Baddeley AD. *The Rivermead Behavioral Memory Test.* Bury St. Edmunds, Thames Valley Test Co.; 1991.

47. Toglia JP. *Contextual Memory Test.* San Antonio, TX, Therapy Skill Builders; 1993.

48. Kopelman M, Wilson, Baddeley AD. *The Autobiographical Memory Interview.* Bury St. Edmonds, Thames Valley Test Co.; 1990.

49. Bennett-Levy J, Powell G. The subjective memory questionnaire (SMQ): An investigation into the self-reporting of "real-life" memory skills. *Br J Soc Clin Psychol.* 1980;19:177-188.

50. Wall N, et al. *Hemiplegic Evaluation.* Boston, Massachusetts Rehabilitation Hospital; 1979.

51. Zoltan B. Visual, visual perceptual and perceptual-motor deficits in brain injured adults: Evaluation, treatment and functional implications. In: Kraft GH, Berrol S. (eds). *Physical Medicine and Rehabilitation Clinics of North America.* Philadelphia, WB Saunders Co.; 1992.

52. Brooks N, Lincoln NB. Assessment for rehabilitation. In: Wilson BA, Moffat N (eds.) *Clinical Management of Memory Problems.* Rockville, MD, Aspen Publishers; 1984.

53. Salmon DP, Butters N. Recent developments in learning and memory: Implications for the rehabili-

tation of the amnesic patient. In: Meir MJ, Benton AL, Diller L. (eds). *Neuropsychological rehabilitation.* New York, Guilford Press; 1987.

54. Freeman MR, Mittenberg W, Dicowden M, Bat-Ami M. Executive and compensatory memory retraining in traumatic brain injury. *Brain Injury.* 1992;6(1):65-70.

55. Glisky EL, Schacter DL. Acquisition of domain-specific knowledge in patients with organic memory disorders. *J of Learning Disabil.* June/July 1988;21(6):333- 351.

56. Zencius A, Wesolowski MD, Burke WH. A comparison of four memory strategies with traumatically brain-injured clients. *Brain Injury.* 1990;4(1):33-38.

57. Atkinson RC, Shiffrin RM. The control of short-term memory. *Sci Am.* 1971;225(2):82-89.

58. Baum B, Hall K. Relationship between constructional praxis and dressing in the head-injured adult. *Am J Occup Ther.* 1981;35(7):438-442.

59. Ben-Yishay Y, et al. *Working Approaches to Remediation of Cognitive Deficits in Brain-damaged Pe. Rehabilitation Monograph 62.* New York, New York University Medical Center, May 1981.

60. Bourne LE, Dominowski RL, Loftus EF. *Cognitive Processes.* Englewood Cliffs, New Jersey, Prentice-Hall, Inc.; 1979.

61. Cook EA, Thigpen R. Identification and management of cognitive and perceptual deficits in the rehabilitation patient. *Rehabilitation Nursing.* Sept/Oct 1993;18(5):3110-3113.

62. Craik F. Human memory. *Ann Rev Psychol.* 1979;30:63-102.

63. Crovitz H. Memory retraining in brain-damaged patients: The airplane list. *Cortex.* 1979;15:131-134.

64. Glasgow RE, Zeiss RA, Barrera JR, Lewinsohn PM. Case studies on remediating memory deficits in brain-damaged individuals. *J Clin Psychol.* 1977;33(4):1049-1054.

65. Harris J. Methods of improving memory. In: Wilson BA, Moffat N (eds.). *Clinical Management of Memory Problems.* Rockville, MD, Aspen Publishers; 1984.

66. Lewinsohn PM, Danaher BG, Kikel S. Visual imagery as a mnemonic aid for brain-injured persons. *J Consult Clin Psychol.* 1977;5(5):717-723.

67. Lezak M. *Neuropsychological Assessment.* New York, Oxford University Press; 1983.

68. Malec J, Questad K. Rehabilitation of memory after craniocerebral trauma: Case report. *Arch Phys Med Rehab.* 1983;64:436-438.

69. Moffat N. Strategies of memory therapy. In: Wilson BA, Moffat N (eds.). *Clinical Management of Memory Problems.* Rockville, MD, Aspen Publishers; 1984.

70. Sandler AB, Harris JL. Use of external memory aids with a head-injured patient. *Amer J Occup Ther.* Feb 1992;46(2):163-1662.

71. Schwartz SM. Adults with traumatic brain injury: Three case studies of cognitive rehabilitation in the home setting. *Amer J Occup Ther.* Jul/Aug 1995;49(7):655-667.

72. Wilson B. Memory therapy in practice. In: Wilson BA, Moffat N (eds.). *Clinical Management of Memory Problems.* Rockville, MD, Aspen Publishers; 1984.

73. Wilson B. Recovery and compensatory strategies in head injured memory impaired people several years after insult. *J Neurol Neurosurg Psychiatry.* Mar 1992;55(3):177-1.

CHAPTER 9

Executive Functions

The T.B.I. or C.V.A. patient often displays deficits in the ability to control impulses, use feedback to control behavior and to evaluate the consequences of his behavior.[1] These problems fall under the category of executive functions. Executive functions are the self-regulating and control functions that direct and organize behavior.[2] Specific component areas include planning, decision making, directed goal selection, self-inhibiting, self-monitoring, self-evaluating, flexible problem solving, initiation and self-awareness.[2-7]

Impaired executive function has been associated with frontal lobe and subcortical limbic system damage.[6,8] It is theorized that the adult level of executive function is reached in three stages.[5] Simple planning and organized visual search develops by age 6, hypothesis testing and impulse control by age 10 and complex motor sequencing and verbal fluency during adolescence.[5] Others have observed that between the age of 1 1/2 and 5 years old and again between ages 5 to 10 years old, a sequence of changes takes place related to a reorganization of attentional, executive and self-reflexive processes.[8]

Ylvisaker and Szekeres describe two categories of executive functions.[6] The first category is knowledge base, which is an organized system of general information, learned skills or routines, rules and procedures. Without this knowledge base, new information is difficult to interpret, organize and remember.

The second system is the executive system and deals with the mental functions related to goal formation, planning and achieving goals.[6] Component areas of this system are "…realistic goal setting (based on an awareness of one's strengths and weaknesses), planning, self-directing and initiating, self-inhibiting, self-monitoring, self-evaluating, self-correcting and flexible problem solving."[6]

Patients with poor executive function are often impulsive, show tangential conversations, perseverative comments and are socially inappropriate.[6] They often cannot adequately monitor the social situation they are in as well as relations with others. These patients will often judge their own performance in general or global terms, rather than looking specifically and objectively at what they have done. When trying to solve a problem, they will only consider one possible solution to a problem and will fail to consider relevant information in choosing the best solutions.

Adequate executive functions allow for effective adaptation and accommodation to changing environmental demands.[4] In order for the patient to reach this level, he must be retrained in awareness of his deficits and learn to control thoughts and actions.[2] It is important to remember that the retraining process should not be so structured that executive activity on the patient's part is no longer required.[6]

The component executive skills of awareness/self-monitoring, planning and organization, problem solving, mental flexibility and initiation are subsequently described in this chapter. Although some associated behavioral issues are discussed, it is not within the scope of this book to cover in detail these areas. The reader is encouraged to search out this information.

Initiation

The C.V.A. or T.B.I. patient may have difficulty in starting a task or activity. The patient may be sitting with a schedule in hand, can give the time, place and name of the therapy, but will remain in his room without cues such as *"Go to your therapy,"* or *"Get started."*[9] Many patients will have good language skills to engage in active conversation but will not initiate it and remain silent until a conversational topic is proposed for them.[6] The patient may lack spontaneity, be slow to respond, and generally show little or no initiative.[10] The patient may be able to plan, organize, and carry out complex tasks, but only when instructed to do so.[10] Often times these behaviors are misinterpreted as intentional lack of motivation or drive.[7]

Recent research has provided hope for the remediation of initiation deficits through incentive training. It is theorized that there are two types of learning: strategy learning and incentive learning.[11] Strategy learning relates to the acquisition and development of "...compensatory behaviors, memory techniques, problem solving methods etc., that the client learns in therapy."[11] Incentive learning on the other hand, is the understanding that the use of a particular strategy in everyday life will result in getting something in return. The patient must apply a given strategy to a real life situation, and get rewarded for using it in order for incentive learning to occur.[11] In three experiments with 24 T.B.I. patients, it was demonstrated that cognitive skills improved immediately and dramatically with the use of incentive training, as long as the therapist created a relevant incentive to activate the patient's performance or initiate the activity.[11] Continued research should indicate what type of incentive is the most effective in eliciting patient initiation.

Evaluation of Initiation

TEST 1: CLINICAL OBSERVATION AND ACTIVITY ANALYSIS

General guidelines for evaluation:
1.   Observe the patient in a number of settings.
2.   Consider the amount of structure and cuing required for initiation of activity by the patient.
3.   Establish functional baseline measures. Consider the frequency and severity of the problem as it relates to function. Select relevant functional areas or tasks as the basis for evaluation and reassessment.

Specific areas and questions to consider and evaluate:
1.   Are there any associated behavioral problems, such as flat or blunted affect? Behavioral outbursts? Disinhibition?

2. Is the patient's behavior generally passive? Does he respond passively to questions or suggestions?
3. What does the patient do during the day? Does someone have to organize his activity for him?
4. What, if any, activities can the patient initiate by himself without cuing or structure?
5. What cuing method or sensory modality appears to be the most effective visual, auditory or tactile kinesthetic cues?
6. Is the patient aware that he has an initiation problem? Does he accept it when it is pointed out to him?
7. Is an associated attentional or memory problem affecting initiation abilities?
    To improve validity, rule out decreased attention, processing, language, apraxia and psychologically based (versus organic) depression as causes of poor performance.

Treatment For Initiation Deficits

Utilizing a Remedial Approach:

1. Provide incentive training as follows:[11]
    a. Monitor the patient's needs and interests in order to identify the most appropriate incentive. Find out what were the patient's pre-morbid interests and motivators.
    b. Make incentives available on an ongoing basis.
    c. Create a training environment where the incentive value is sufficient to elicit appropriate levels of interest and performance.
    d. Teach strategies to the point where they become habitual.
    e. Provide an opportunity for incentive learning by allowing the patient to use newly learned strategies in a context which will provide rewards, ie, money, social praise, movie, dinner out, etc.
2. Provide sensory input (visual, auditory, kinesthetic and tactile) to elicit a motor output (initiation). For example, tactile and kinesthetic stimulation of the patient's arm combined with verbal cuing may be utilized to cue the patient to initiate upper extremity dressing.
3. Apply concepts from the Affolter approach. Provide nonverbal tactile-kinesthetic guiding to assist the patient in initiating the activity.

Utilizing an Adaptive Approach:

1. Provide signals such as alarm watches to trigger an activity.[6]
2. Utilize an audio cassette which can be turned on by someone else with step by step instructions to follow. For example, *"Take your medicine, open the little one with the white cap, take two white pills, drink some water, etc."*[9]
3. Assist the patient in developing an awareness of the problem so that he can begin to develop his own internal cuing system for initiating tasks.

Self-Monitoring/Awareness

The patient who has sustained brain damage often has poor awareness or insight into the limitations associated with his disorder. A patient may be totally unaware of blatant deficits that are obvious to those around him. Some patients deny that they have a problem, to the point of becoming hostile to those who attempt to point deficits out. Still others may be indifferent to their limitations. Other patients may exhibit complete denial and resort to fabrication when someone is pointing out a deficit area.

Decreased awareness is an inability to recognize deficits or problem circumstances caused by neurological injury.[12] There is a failure to acknowledge impairments of cognitive and/or motor function when questioned.[13,14] Recent research has indicated that an unawareness of cognitive deficits does not always coincide with unawareness of motor deficits.[13,14] Areas which have been found to influence awareness include memory or intellectual impairments, decreased sensory and perceptual abilities, decreased inhibition and inpulsivity or inability to plan for the future.[12]

Decreased awareness of deficits can have a profound effect on the patient's behavior as well as his ability to participate in rehabilitation.[13,15-18] In some cases, the individual will not seek out or accept treatment.[16,18] Prigatano et al,[16] in a study of head injured patients, discovered that patients underestimated their abilities in emotional and social interactions. These patients had difficulty in handling arguments, adjusting to unexpected changes and controlling their temper. These skills are all required for social competence.

One can view decreased awareness at two levels: 1) unawareness of the deficit itself and 2) unawareness of the consequences of the deficit. Prigatano[18] has identified two types of deficits depending on the location of brain damage. Pre-frontal brain damage can cause poor self-awareness, about social judgment, the ability to anticipate change, or decreased interpersonal awareness. Decreased awareness exhibited by parietal lobe damage on the other hand, involves awareness of body image, perceptual, sensory and motor abilities. Different evaluation tools may help delineate these different aspects of unawareness.

Barco et al[12] identify three levels of awareness which can serve as a basis for evaluation and treatment. These areas are defined by Barco et al[12] as follows:

1. Intellectual Awareness—the cognitive capacity of the client to understand to some degree that a particular function is diminished from pre-morbid levels
2. Emergent Awareness—the ability of clients to recognize a problem when it is actually occurring
3. Anticipation Awareness—the ability to anticipate that a problem is going to happen because of some deficit

Some degree of intellectual awareness is considered to be a pre-requisite for both emergent and anticipatory awareness. Patients with poor emergent awareness can describe their deficit and what they should do for it, however, because they don't recognize that a problem is occurring, they cannot compensate when necessary. The complete understanding of the implications of one's deficits is the highest level of intellectual awareness, and is closely linked with anticipatory awareness.[12]

Functional implications of decreased awareness include impulsiveness and poor safety awareness. The patient must be taught to control and monitor his performance and how to use feedback effectively.[19] The patient often has low frustration tolerance often resulting in anger.[20] The patient will be unable to correct any errors or mistakes because he is unable to perceive them.[10] As previously noted, some patients may be able to perceive their errors but are unable to self-correct, and regulate the quality of their behavior and performance. This deficit of poor self-monitoring is the inability to evaluate and regulate the quality of our behavior.[2] This inability to control and monitor behavior will in turn affect judgment in all functional tasks. The patient, for example, may impulsively try to get out of bed and walk to the bathroom despite paralysis, or he may be unsafe around the stove.

Due to the documented occurrence of decreased awareness in brain-damaged patients and associated functional implications, evaluation is crucial to patient management and treatment planning decisions. Its evaluation can assist in providing the patient's family with necessary education, support, management strategies and the assistance in the development of realistic goals.[15]

Evaluation of Decreased Awareness

TEST 1: CLINICAL OBSERVATION AND ACTIVITY ANALYSIS

General guidelines for evaluation:
1. Determine whether the patient is aware of and responsive to his environment. One measure of the patient's awareness is his ability to utilize feedback.[21]
2. Observe if the patient requests clarification of instructions appropriately and attempts to self-correct. Try to elicit this response by giving unclear or hasty directions or by giving too much information.
3. Observe the patient in a number of settings and activities during the day. Limited insight, poor safety awareness, and impulsiveness can vary depending on the setting and the task. Define what types of conditions (including specific instructions to inhibit a certain behavior) improve or worsen disinhibited or socially inappropriate behavior.[6]
4. Establish functional baseline measures. Consider the degree and frequency of the problem. Select relevant functional tasks as the basis of evaluation and reassessment.

Specific areas and questions to consider and evaluate:
1. Can the patient perceive and verbalize (or somehow communicate) the extent and type of problems he is having?
2. Is he willing to try to understand and accept his problems when they are pointed out to him?
3. Once he admits that he has a specific problem, can he then perceive how it will affect his overall function beyond a specific task?
4. How does the environment affect the patient's awareness and behavior? Does a quiet structured environment decrease impulsivity and increase insight? In which environments does safety become an issue, eg, kitchen, community?
5. Does verbal, visual, or tactile cuing improve insight or decrease impulsiveness?
6. What is the duration and frequency of the patient's impulsiveness and decreased insight or safety awareness?
7. Is there a task or tasks that are particularly helpful in illustrating a specific problem to the patient?

Scoring:
Nonstandardized.
These and similar questions can be incorporated into a checklist or used in conjection with a frequency rating scale (eg, always/sometimes/rarely/never).
To improve validity, rule out decreased attention, poor memory, and aphasia as causes of poor performance.

TEST 2: SELF-AWARENESS QUESTIONNAIRE[15]*

Description:
This is a 27-item orientation and awareness questionnaire.
All orientation questions and three of the four awareness-of-brain-injury questions have a three choice format. Present verbally all three choices and then repeating all choices until one response is affirmed. All other items are yes/no questions.

Self-Awareness Questionnaire

Orientation to time and place
(Three choice format)
Day
Month
Date
Year
Town
What is this place?
(army)   (school)   (rehabilitation center)
What is the name of this place?

Awareness of brain injury (personalize these items for each survivor)
What happened to you to bring you here?
(parents/relatives sent you here)   (car accident/fall/blow)*   (volunteered to come)
Why are you here?
(to receive therapy)   (punishment)   (unsure)
Has your brain been injured?   (Yes)   (No)
When were you injured?
(at birth)   (I have not been injured)   (actual year)*

Awareness of physical impairment
Can you walk?   (Yes)   (No)
Do you have difficulty moving your legs?   (Yes)   (No)
Can you move both your arms normally?   (Yes)   (No)
Do you have difficulty moving your fingers?   (Yes)   (No)

Awareness of communication impairment
Can you speak normally?   (Yes)   (No)
Can you understand what people say to you?   (Yes)   (No)
Do you have difficulty reading?   (Yes)   (No)
Do you have difficulty writing?   (Yes)   (No)

Activities of daily living
Do you need help to feed yourself?   (Yes)   (No)
Can you dress yourself?   (Yes)   (No)
Do you need help to bathe yourself?   (Yes)   (No)
Can you shave/apply makeup yourself?   (Yes)   (No)

Awareness of sensory/cognitive deficits
Do you have a good memory?   (Yes)   (No)
Do you have good vision?   (Yes)   (No)
Do you get fatigued/tired easily?   (Yes)   (No)
Do you have trouble thinking clearly?   (Yes)   (No)

---

*Reproduced with permission from Aspen Publishers, 200 Orchard Ridge Dr., Gaithersburg, MD.

TEST 3: EVALUATION OF THREE LEVELS OF AWARENESS[12]

General guidelines for evaluation:[12]

1. Intellectual Awareness—evaluated through informal interview. Ask the patient to describe what difficulties he is having since his injury or the onset of disease. Can the patient describe the functional implications these deficits have on his life?

2. Emergent Awareness—evaluated through clinical observation during a cognitive task or functional activity. Does the patient recognize and correct problems? Does the patient become frustrated with the task, but is unable to understand what is causing the frustration? Upon questioning, is the patient accurately able to reflect on how he is doing?

3. Anticipatory Awareness—evaluated through clinical observation combined with timed questions. For example, ask, What types of problems, if any, you might expect to have in (a variety of situations) and why do you think you will have a problem in that situation? Don't provide cuing or assistance to the patient during clinical observation of anticipatory awareness because you have to observe what the patient initiates on his own to see if anticipatory awareness does exist.

Treatment of Decreased Awareness

Utilizing a Remedial Approach:

1. Intellectual Awareness
   - Without at least a minimal amount of intellectual awareness, a remedial approach is not appropriate.[12]
   - If there is a minimal amount of intellectual awareness, provide immediate, objective and concrete feedback to the patient during activities.
   - Have the patient make a strengths and weaknesses list and show to the therapist.

2. Emergent Awareness
   - Provide feedback to the patient during and after a task. Use consistent cuing or terminology and be direct and very specific. Feedback should specify the problem as it occurs and explain what the observable signs are of how the problem is affecting performance.
   - Have the patient do a self-rating scale for specific problems. The patient and therapist (or family) can do the rating concurrently. The goal over time is for the patient and therapist ratings to be similar. Use the ratings after treatment session is over and discuss the results with the patient.

3. Anticipatory Awareness
   - Guide the patient into planning for deficits. In other words, cue the patient to plan and anticipate what deficits may affect performance before starting a task. Reduce cuing as the patient becomes more aware.

4. Utilize videotaping, role playing and group treatment techniques as appropriate to the patient's level of awareness. For example, use simulated social situations when teaching patient social skills.[22] Teach the patient strategies for dealing with anger. Practice sessions in dealing with a hierarchy of anger situations.[20] Have the patient practice positive self-verbalizations.

5. Reward the patient not just for completing a goal but for accurate prediction of how and if he can complete the goal.[6]

6. Utilize "activity processing" as follows:[23]
   - Reiterate the purpose of what you're doing.
   - Identify with the patient what are the performance boundaries, skills and limitations of performance.
   - Discuss successful strategies as well as performance barriers.
   - Relate the treatment experience to relevant home or work tasks.
   - Collaborate with the patient on new goals based on performance and activity processing discussion.
7. Utilize self-evaluation forms.* For example, when working on social awareness, the following could be used with the patient:

Self-Evaluation
Social Interaction Incident
1. What happened?
2. How did it make me feel?
3. What did I do?
4. How did that make _____ feel?
5. Could I have behaved differently?
6. Could _____ have behaved differently?
7. Could I have avoided the situation?
8. What might be another way to handle the situation in the future?

Self-evaluation forms should be used in incidents when the patient handled an interaction well, not just when there was a problem. Reward the patient for the self-evaluation process even if the original need for filling out the form was due to inappropriate behavior.

Utilizing an Adaptive Approach:

1. Intellectual Awareness

Provide repetitive education to the patient and his family regarding the patient's decreased awareness and how it will affect function. Focus also on brain function and types of damage that can occur.

Provide external environmental modifications and cuing as needed. Special care should be taken for activities where safety is an issue, ie, kitchen, ambulation, driving.

2. Emergent Awareness

Utilize "situational compensation."[12] This is compensation that is triggered by a particular situation. Therapist identifies the situation, develops an appropriate compensation plan and trains the patient in its use through practice and repetition. For example, the patient has the

---

*Self-monitoring improves with self-instruction because the auditory feedback allows the patient to monitor errors more frequently.[33]

intellectual awareness to know the house needs cleaning, but not sufficient emergent awareness of how to go about cleaning it. A checklist of household tasks may be developed and provided to the patient to help him compensate.

3. Anticipatory Awareness

Provide recognition compensations.[12] When the patient recognizes a problem is occurring, this recognition cues him to initiate a compensation strategy. The therapist helps the patient to develop a strategy. If the patient is already using a strategy, the therapist should evaluate its effectiveness and modify it as needed. Utilize the patient's strengths when teaching the compensation strategy.

Planning and Organization

The ability to learn and achieve any goal necessitates organization and planning. In order to formulate a goal, the individual must be able to determine what he needs and wants, and foresee the future realization of these needs.[24,25] The determination and organization of the steps needed to achieve a goal involve several component skills of planning. In order to plan, the individual must be able to conceptualize change from the present situation, relate objectively to the environment, conceive alternatives, weigh alternatives and make a choice, and develop a structure or framework to give direction to the carrying out of the plan.[10]

Disorders of planning and organization are generally associated with frontal lobe dysfunction and should be distinguished from memory, attentional and mental flexibility deficits.[26,27] The ability to form and shift concepts allows for flexible planning. Impaired abstraction and mental flexibility, therefore, will adversely affect planning ability.[27] In addition, if the patient is unable to organize information in order to facilitate learning and recall, the information may be stored but in a scattered manner.[26] If the information is less accessible for retrieval, then the patient's problems may be erroneously interpreted as a memory problem.

Processing strategies are crucial to effective planning and organization. These strategies can be defined as "…organized approaches, routines or tactics that operate to select and guide the processing of information."[28] In order to develop good processing strategies, the patient must be able to estimate the degree of task difficulty. If the patient understands and realistically interprets task difficulty, then an appropriate plan or strategy can be developed. If this understanding or awareness is lacking, then the patient's strategies will be ineffective.

The patient with a planning deficit may in fact lack the foresight and sustained attention necessary for achieving a desired goal. Often the patient can describe in detail the elements in planning and organizing personal events, but show poor, unrealistic or illogical plans for himself.[10,29] If asked to write a description of a familiar activity for example, the patient may list a series of unrelated features because he neglected to create a plan for the description from the beginning.[6]

Evaluation of Planning and Organization

TEST 1: CLINICAL OBSERVATION AND ACTIVITY ANALYSIS

General guidelines for evaluation:

1. Determine whether the patient is aware that he has a planning deficit. Defective planning often can be revealed by asking the patient what he intends to do.
2. Observe the patient in a number of settings and activities during the day. Can the patient plan for activities requiring two step operations? Three step? More complex operations?
3. Give the patient a complex task without instruction. If the patient begins the task without a plan, ask him to create one and begin the task again. The patient's plan can then be evaluated for organization and completeness.[6]
4. Establish functional baseline measures. Consider the duration and frequency of the problem. Select relevant functional tasks as the basis of evaluation and reassessment.

Specific areas and questions to consider and evaluate:[30,31]

1. Is the patient logical and consistent in his approach to the task?
2. How reliable is his chosen method?
3. Is there a common problem or consistently faulty planning strategy that is generalized to several activities?
4. Can the patient conceptualize change (as evidenced through verbal or other means of communication) from the present?
5. Can the patient present alternatives to an established plan?
6. Can he weigh these alternatives and make a choice based on his judgments?
7. Does he appear to have a framework for the plan or direction he is demonstrating for task completion?
8. Can he accurately estimate task difficulty?

Note: Questions and observations such as these can be applied to both functional and cognitive perceptual motor tasks. For example, inability to complete block designs (refer to Test 1 in the section on Problem Solving) and layout of graphic designs can be indicative or poor planning and task organization.

Scoring:

Nonstandardized. These and similar questions can be incorporated into a checklist or used in conjunction with a frequency rating scale (eg, always/sometimes/rarely/never).

To improve validity, rule out decreased attention, poor memory, decreased mental flexibility and abstraction, impaired problem solving and aphasia as causes of poor performance.

Treatment of Planning and Organization Deficits

Utilizing a Remedial Approach:

1. Teach the patient to attend to the organizational structure of information he is to learn. For example, to outline prose material and divide into categories when learning it.[26]
2. Have the patient verbalize, if possible, a plan before, during and after a given activity. Gradually fade out overt verbalizations.[32] Also have the patient estimate task difficulty and predict the outcome of his identified plan.[7] Have the patient evaluate the accuracy of predictions.[2]
3. Research has indicated that training in plan-ahead and self-verbalization strategies is effective in remediating planning disorders following a T.B.I. or C.V.A.[1,32,33] Self-verbalization requires the patient to sequence each step of the task before beginning. Three examples of

self-questioning techniques are described:

    a.   What do I need to do?

        I need to . . . . .

        What do I need to do now?

        I need to . . . . .

        What do I need to do now?

        I need to . . . . .

    b.   What is it I want to accomplish?

        What changes need to occur to move from the present situation to my desired goal?

        What are the possible ways to make the necessary changes?

        What is the sequence or order of steps required to make the changes?

        Are there any alternatives to my plan? Which is the best alternative to use to reach my goal?

        How will I know that I have reached my goal and that my plan was successful?

    c.   What is my goal?

        What is the purpose of my goal?

        Where will I perform the activity?

        How long will it take?

        What materials do I need?

        What is the order of the steps I need to take?

        Will I be able to reach my goal?

        How will I track my progress?

As the patient asks these questions of himself, he can jot down his ideas or thought processes as an additional cuing mechanism. Analysis of this written plan by the therapist can then be utilized to identify any faulty planning or judgments. The patient then is encouraged to develop alternative strategies.

4.   Incorporate questioning techniques in a variety of tasks and settings. For example, searching tasks can be utilized.[6] Establish a search plan with the patient by asking the following questions:[6]

    a.   What are we looking for? (object of the search)

        Where do you suppose it is? (location, goal)

        How can we find it? (plan)

        How much time do we have to look? (time frame)

        Do you think we can find it? (prediction of success)

Utilizing an Adaptive Approach:

1.   Provide daily reminders, appointment calendars and to do lists for the patient. Provide not just what the patient needs to do but what he needs to do to complete the task.[2]

2.   Identify peak performance times and try to have these times as uninterrupted as possible.[2]

Try to schedule important tasks during this time.
3. Provide written and/or verbal step-by-step instructions for task completion. Identify which tasks are crucial to the patient's occupational function.
4. Educate the family about the patient's planning and organization deficit and how to compensate for it in the home and community.

Problem Solving

Problem solving is not a single function, but rather the integration of several cognitive skills. It requires attention, the ability to devise and initiate a plan, information access (both sensory from the environment and memory) and a feedback system, which gives information on the effectiveness of the solution and the need for revision.[34-37] Additional prerequisites for problem solving include good impulse control, the ability to organize and categorize, mental flexibility, and reasoning skills.[38] Problem solving is an active process and breakdown can occur at any stage. In addition, the patient's reasoning ability can determine the quality of the manner in which a problem will be formulated and the strategies applied for problem solutions.[38]

Effective problem solving involves some initial understanding of the problem. How good this initial representation is will determine how quickly an accurate solution can be formulated. Motivation can affect both the perception of a problem and whether or not a solution is attempted. Motivation problems can originate from depression and/or decreased self-awareness of deficits.[38] Problem solving can vary, depending on whether the patient has access to and utilizes a memory aid, for instance.[34] Approaching a problem and comparing past and present experiences through memory skills enable an individual to think in an orderly manner.[39,40] The individual must be able to screen out and discard irrelevant information.[41-43] Problem solving ability will be affected if adequate attention is not taken to analyze the stimulus problem or situation completely.[44] Once the information is registered and screened, the individual must be able to modify, transform, and organize it to come up with a solution.[34,35] Problem solving requires mental flexibility. The individual needs to be able to reformulate initial ideas when a solution is incorrect or fails to solve the problem.[36] Finally, the individual must be able to make judgments about the quality of potential solutions.[34]

Adamovich[44] describes four theoretical thinking processes involved in problem solving. The patient must first recognize and analyze relevant and missing information (convergent thinking). Next, he must draw conclusions about a given situation, based on certain principles, in a systematic manner (deductive reasoning). The patient must then formulate a solution based on details that lead to a standard conclusion (inductive reasoning). Finally, the patient must be able to generate abstract concepts which deviate from standard concepts. Lezak[10] identifies four stages of executive functions in problem solving as follows:

1. Goal formation—What do I want or need?
2. Planning—How will I get what I need?
3. Carrying out activities—Am I doing things to reach my goal?
4. Effective performance—Are my activities fulfilling my objective?

Ben-Yishay and Diller[45] support both Adamovich and Lezak in their model of problem solving. They describe an eight-stage model of problem solving which incorporates some convergent, divergent and executive stages. The eight stages are outlined as follows:

1. Formulate problem
2. Analyze conditions of problem
3. Formulate strategy and plan of action
4. Choose the relevant tactics (apply skills, prioritize)
5. Execute plan—self-monitor operation
6. Compare solution against problem
7. Satisfaction and closure
8. Integration into attitudes and skills and personalize (what does it mean to me?).

Ben-Yishay and Diller[45] also include in their theoretical framework for treatment the concept of two domains of skills in the problem solving process. These two domains are: 1) the core skills which include skills such as attention, sensation, tone, language, or memory, and 2) the two higher domains of problem solving/rational processes and emotive, imaginative and emphatic processes. They theorize that disorders of high domains can be caused by the core deficits and that effective problem solving depends on the interaction between the two domains. Evaluation and treatment, they believe, should address all aspects of the eight-stage process and domains of skills.

The patient with problem solving deficits may exhibit concrete thinking, impulsivity, confusion as to where to start solving a problem, difficulty sequencing information, and trouble learning from mistakes as well as successes.[46,47] Unless the patient has some degree of problem solving skills, he will be unable to apply newly learned skills to new situations.[48] The clinical manifestations of poor problem solving can reflect a breakdown in any aspect or stage of the overall process previously outlined. The evaluation of problem solving therefore can "…be facilitated by utilizing a variety of traditional and non-traditional measures as well as a detailed process analysis of the underlying deficit."[38]

Evaluation of Problem Solving

TEST 1: COGNITIVE STRATEGIES — BLOCK DESIGN[49]*

Description:
The patient is asked to reproduce a block design that the examiner has constructed. While the patient is performing the task, the evaluator records his progression of attempts on the cognitive strategies worksheet (Figure 9-1).

Scoring:
Nonstandardized.
Intact: The patient approaches the problem in a meaningful organized way and evaluates his solution in comparison with the stimulus.
Impaired: The patient's approach is disorganized (trial and error); he is unable to make comparisons and judgments about the solution and the stimulus.
To improve validity, rule out spatial neglect and constructional apraxia as a cause of poor performance.

---

*Cognitive Strategies worksheet adapted and reproduced with permission from Santa Clara Valley Medical Center, San Jose, CA.

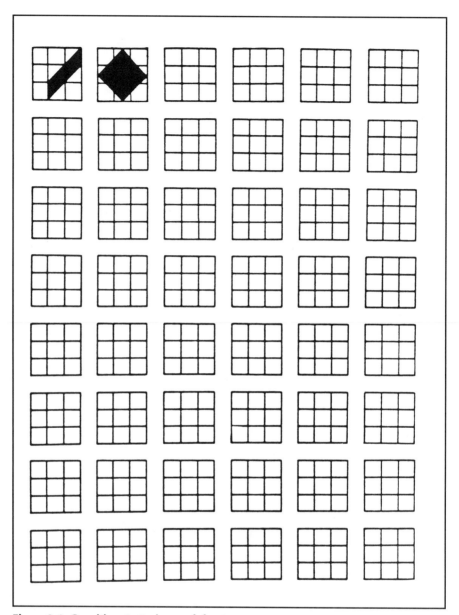

Figure 9-1. Cognitive strategies worksheet.

Note: the examiner is focusing not on whether the patient can complete the task, but rather on how he completes it or attempts to complete it.

TEST 2: CLINICAL OBSERVATIONS AND ACTIVITY ANALYSIS[10,34]*

Description:
Provide an unstructured task without guidance from the therapist. Observe for the following abilities. Problem solving is divided into three stages: preparation, production, and judgment. Clinical observations in selected activities are based on questions related to these three stages as follows:

---

*Adapted and reproduced with permission from Prentice-Hall, Inc., Englewood Cliffs, NJ.

1. Preparation and understanding the problem (problem analysis)
   a. Can the patient identify any or all elements of the problem?
   b. Can the patient identify solution criteria?
   c. Can the patient identify any limitations or constraints related to potential attempts at problem solving?
   d. Can he describe or indicate how the problem compares with those he has already solved?
   e. Can the patient divide the problem into parts or components?
   f. Can the patient construct a simple problem by ignoring some information?
2. Production: generating possible solutions
   a. Can the patient retrieve necessary information from long-term memory?
   b. Can or does the patient scan the environment for available information?
   c. Can or does the patient operate or act on the content in short-term memory?
   d. Can or does the patient store information in long-term memory for later use?
   e. Can the patient generate a potential solution?
3. Judgment: evaluating the solutions generated
   a. Does the patient compare the generated solution with the initial solution criteria?
   b. Does the patient decide either that the problem as been solved or that more work is needed?

Scoring:
Nonstandardized. The preceding or similar questions can be incorporated into a yes/no checklist or related to a frequency rating scale.
To improve validity, rule out poor attention, memory, impulsiveness or other factors as causes of poor performance.

Treatment of Problem Solving Deficits
Utilizing a Remedial Approach:

1. Train the patient in developing the following skills:[50]
   a. The ability to recognize at a general level that a given task or situation is a problem for which a solution is not yet available.
   b. Have the patient read and reread directions and ask questions to help his understanding of the problem.
   c. Have the patient describe in his own words the main points, discriminating between the facts and opinions or assumptions.
   d. Train the patient to identify problem solving goals, restraints and circumstances that cause the task to be problematic.
   e. Train the patient to generate alternatives or potential solutions to the problem.
   f. Teach the patient to evaluate the alternative solutions and to select the most effective one. Ask the patient why he came up with a given solution and decided the potential consequences.
   g. Train the patient to recognize "faulty" paths, correct errors and return to the original hypothesis.*

---

*Research utilizing this specific remedial approach indicated improved problem solving after three months.

2. Utilize problem solving worksheets such as the following:[51]

Activity: Yellow Pages[52]*

Purpose:
1. Improve problem-solving skills.
2. Improve ability to make logical deductions.
3. Improve speed in decision making.

Supplies:
Trial/Score Sheets #1 - #5, a copy of the written instructions for these Trials, pencil, Yellow Pages, Answer Key, Therapist Observation Sheet, Weekly Performance Summary, White Self-Assessment Quiz, stopwatch (optional).

Activity Description/Session Strategies
For each Trial, the client is given ten hypothetical problems or situations that might require contacting local places of business. Using the Yellow Pages, the client must record in the space provided on the Trial Sheet, the name of the business and telephone number that logically address each situation. The client receives verbal instructions supplemented by written instructions. A Demonstration Item is included in each Trial to be used at the therapist's discretion.

The client should be instructed to review his work with the therapist after finishing each Trial. The Answer Key provides possible headings under which appropriate businesses might be located for each item and is intended to be used by the patient and therapist during the review process. After reviewing the Trial, the patient completes the White Self-Assessment Quiz and compares it with the therapist's version. The client and therapist discuss and determine strategy modifications for subsequent Trials.

Speed in decision making is an important component in this exercise and should be emphasized. Some clients may waste time reading advertisements, or, for example, looking unnecessarily for the dry cleaner closest to their home rather than recording the answer that they locate first. When it is evident that the patient is becoming distracted to components of the task itself, the therapist may opt to time each Trial in order to graphically demonstrate the effect of this problem on performance.

Written Instruction:
1. Before you begin work, you will need to make sure that you have a pencil, a Yellow Pages directory and a Trial Sheet and that you know where to locate the Answer Key.
2. Beginning with item "A," you are to read the hypothetical problem or situation that might require you to contact a local place of business.
3. Using the Yellow Pages, you are to record (in the space provided) the name of a business and telephone number that logically address the situation.

---

*Reproduced with permission from Aspen Publications, Gaithersburg, MD.

4. After completing item "J", bring your Trial Sheet to the therapist. Using the Answer Key, discuss your answers with him and together determine whether or not you have made errors.
5. Next, request the White Self-Assessment Quiz and fill it out.
6. After filling out the Quiz, be prepared to discuss the results with the therapist.

Resources: The Telephone
Yellow Pages

Trial #2

Date:

Name:

Demonstration Task

Your carpet needs to be cleaned.

Answer: Carpet & Rug Cleaners: (Therapist provides example).

A. You have some money to invest.

_____

B. You are hungry for a chocolate-covered doughnut.

_____

C. You want to have your hair colored.

_____

D. You want to buy a baseball bat.

_____

E. Your toilet is backed up.

_____

F. You would like to have someone answer your telephone calls.

_____

G. You need a water softener.

_____

H. Your washing machine needs to be repaired.

_____

I. Your lawn needs to be fertilized.

_____

J. You want to have a picture framed.

_____

Accuracy (number of errors):   _____

3. Teach the patient to utilize "chaining" of the activity, ie, breaking it down into functional components.

   a. Have the patient describe how he would define and carry out a given problem.[40] Have him continue the process by describing how he is doing something as he is doing it.[29] Progress from external environmental cues to internal cues by subvocalization (ie, the patient tells himself what he is doing as he is doing it).

   b. Have the patient plan the step in problem solution before doing it.

   c. Have the patient label the steps of the task to make them more meaningful, thus increasing his memory of them.[29]

4. Have the patient perform a variety of tasks in a number of settings, utilizing the remedial techniques just described.

Treatment could focus both on tabletop and functional activities. For example: Try cognitive flexibility worksheets that alternate between subtraction and addition and link these with counting change and money handling. Combining the approaches could improve motivation because the patient learns the relevance of the skills to ADL.

Utilizing an Adaptive Approach:

1. Monitor how the task or environment can be altered in order to improve problem solving skills. Provide adaptations as needed.

   a. Provide external cues to reduce the patient's use of inappropriate strategies.[46]

   b. Instruct the patient to check for errors before proceeding.

   When giving external cues, remember that you know how to solve the problem and the patient may not.[34] Make sure that the connection between the cue and the solution is clear. Ask yourself, "How will the patient use this cue?"

2. Identify key areas of occupational performance that are affected by impaired problem solving. For the targeted areas, provide step-by-step instructions for task completion.

3. Teach the patient the importance of asking for help when he is unable to solve a given problem. Practice this skill with the patient through role playing and community re-integration treatment.

4. Apply concepts from a dynamic interactional approach: utilize patient questioning techniques to identify the strategy use (conceptual characteristic) the patient is utilizing. Provide feedback to the patient for faulty strategies. Identify effective strategies and provide opportunities for the patient to utilize these strategies in a number of contexts (multicontext).

Mental Flexibility and Abstraction

Many patients who have sustained a C.V.A. or T.B.I. have difficulty in conceptual thinking. A concrete attitude is common in which experiences, objects, and behavior are all interpreted by the patient at the most obvious concrete value.[10] The patient with poor mental flexibility will have difficulty developing concepts and being able to respond to shifting demands of a situation.[53] The patient is unable to change strategies or details of a task performance when the circumstances change or there is an error.[54] The deficit is characterized by an inefficient use of

available processing ability.[55] Some theorize that this ability is related to controlled information processing rather than automatic processing.[55]

The patient with poor mental flexibility will have difficulty releasing a particular stimulus
from his attention. The patient's behavior appears perseverative and an appropriate set of
responses may be followed by a set of inappropriate responses. This occurs because the patient
continues to respond to prior cues that are no longer relevant.[29,56] The patient may show poor
association ability and have difficulty in evaluating the relevance of the result obtained from a
given problem.[35] This stimulus-bound or perseverative behavior makes it difficult for the
patient to generalize knowledge for future problem solution.

Impaired abstraction is a related, commonly occurring deficit exhibited by the C.V.A. or
T.B.I. patient.[57] Patients with poor abstraction have limited imagination and stick to people,
objects and events that catch their eye at once.[50] These patients fail to form concepts or generalize from individual events, fail to plan ahead, and are unable to go beyond the immediate
stimulus situation.[58] The patient is unable to analyze the relationship between objects and their
properties.[38]

Some researchers consider memory deficits as a partial cause of concrete thinking.[39,59]
Severe anterograde amnesia in cases of head injury is associated with subtle or severe problems
with abstraction and decreased "mental flexibility," which in turn results in the patient's inability to learn and integrate new information for future conceptualization.[59] Theoretically, patients
with poor abstraction and decreased mental flexibility are unable to perceive similarities and
differences or to identify the important features in objects and events, because they are unable
to keep these objects and events in mind.[39] Owing to a memory deficit, they are unable to make
comparisons or are unable to retain the comparisons they have already made.

Evaluation of Mental Flexibility

TEST 1: ODD-EVEN CROSS-OUT[29]

Description:
This task tests the patient's ability to shift from one task to another. The patient is provided with a visual search worksheet with a series of numbers on it. He is asked to begin crossing out all the even numbers, and partially through the task is asked to cross out only the
odd numbers. This instruction is subsequently reversed back to the even numbers, then back
to the odd, and so on.

Scoring:
Nonstandardized.
Intact — The patient is able to shift back and forth (odd-even) on all occasions as request-
ed by the therapist.
Impaired — The patient is able to shift back and forth (odd-even) for only a portion of the
task.
Unable — The patient is unable to successfully make the switch.
To improve validity, rule out decreased attention, decreased comprehension, visual neglect,
visual field deficits, and decreased visual scanning as causes of poor performance.

TEST 2: DYNAMIC INTERACTIONAL ASSESSMENT

Description:
Please refer to Test 2, Dynamic Interactional Assessment and Table 8-2 for a description.

Evaluation of Abstraction

TEST 1: CONCEPT FORMATION AND ABSTRACTION[35]
Concept formation involves the ability to define objects, compare and differentiate, establish logical relationships and categorize. The following sample questions illustrate the evaluation of each of these components of concept formation and abstraction.[35]

1. Definition-abstraction. The patient is asked to define a specific word, eg, chair, apple.

Scoring:
Nonstandardized. The therapist notes how the patient makes use of abstract categories.

2. Comparison-differentiation. The patient is asked to relate a pair of ideas through:
    a. Common ground, eg, refrigerator and stove, dresser and sofa.
    b. Differences, eg, the difference between a fox and a dog, or a bed and a chair.

Scoring:
Nonstandardized. The therapist notes whether the patient is able to identify similarities and differences between the paired ideas presented.

3. Logical relationships. The patient is asked to relate a word to a given series, eg, a dog is an _____, a knife is a _____.

Scoring:
Nonstandardized. The therapist notes the patient's ability to establish logical relationships through completion of the series presented.

4. Opposites. The patient is asked to supply the opposite of the word the therapist gives him, eg, high-low, tall-short.

Scoring:
Nonstandardized. The therapist notes the patient's ability to supply the opposite.

5. Categories. The patient is asked to identify the word that does not belong in a series of words the therapist provides, eg, father, mother, brother, sister, friend.

Scoring:
Nonstandardized. The therapist notes the patient's ability to identify the word that does not belong in the series.
To improve validity, rule out decreased attention, memory and aphasia (especially comprehension) as causes of poor performance.

Treatment For Mental Flexibility and Abstraction
Utilizing a Remedial Approach:

1. Have the patient perform tabletop activities that require numerous mental shifts and variations within the task, eg, tasks involving shifting from color to the written word, or the substitution of visual instructions for verbal instructions.

2. Utilize computer training with software designed specifically for the remediation of deficits of mental flexibility.

Utilizing an Adaptive Approach:

1. If the patient is unable to abstract, teach the patient how to make greater use of his concrete thinking skills in problem solving.[38]
2. Utilizing a functional approach, ask the patient to perform, for example, a kitchen task that includes hot and cold meal preparation and functional categorization. Observe whether the patient can shift and organize his behavior within the overall activity. Provide cuing when necessary to compensate for the impaired mental flexibility or abstraction to increase the patient's independence.
3. Apply concepts from a dynamic interactional approach by altering task demands (surface characteristics) and type and amount of feedback for mental shifting between stimulus depending on the patient's performance.
4. Utilize external aids such as written or audiotape instructions for relevant areas of function to compensate for the deficit.
5. Teach the patient and his family about the deficit and how it will affect his daily life.

Generalization and Transfer

Although the terms generalization and transfer are often used interchangeably, they are actually two separate concepts. Transfer of learning involves training skills which are applicable in specific situations.[57] It relates the effect of training specific skills and the extent to which these abilities facilitate or limit new learning.[11] Modern theories of transfer of learning focus on the concept of the "problem space", or similarity of cognitive processing demands common to two tasks.[11] It is believed positive transfer will occur when the patient uses the same knowledge in a similar way in successive tasks. It is also assumed positive transfer occurs only as long as the same training is used in the same way across a sequence of tasks. Hypothetically, two types of learning can transfer: declarative (the patient's existing storehouse of knowledge) and procedural (a specific skill that may apply in only one situation).[11]

The patient's ability to transfer new learning can change through the course of treatment due to spontaneous neurological recovery and therefore needs to be evaluated on an ongoing basis.[60]

As described in Chapter 1, the surface characteristics of a given task will dictate the amount of transfer of learning that is required. The adaptive approach with direct treatment in ADL, for example, requires only near transfer.[60] Transfer of learning from remedial cognitive and perceptual tasks will have more than three to six surface characteristics which differ from functional tasks, and would therefore require intermediate transfer.[60] Some theorize that in addition to surface characteristics of a task affecting transfer, the way in which the patient learns to organize the task is a predictor of how much transfer will occur.[61] It is recommended, therefore, that the therapist show the patient how the organization applies in a variety of different settings. If the patient does not understand how a given strategy or organization applies to everyday life, then transfer will be minimal.

Generalization involves the ability to use a newly learned strategy in a novel situation.[57] The therapist can increase the amount of generalization by varying the task elements while simultaneously keeping the organization relatively constant.[11] The patient will therefore begin to understand how the same organizational technique can apply in a variety of settings. Successful generalization provides the patient with the adaptability to perform correctly across a variety of environments and tasks, as well as the ability to perform tasks without need for further instruction.[62]

Evaluation of Generalization and Transfer

TEST 1: MODIFICATION OF ADL[60]

Description:
Modify ADL treatment from one day to the next at the beginning of treatment. For example, modify the surface characteristics during dressing training. One day place all clothes out in an organized manner and the next place them on the bed in a haphazard manner. Watch for the patient's response.

Scoring:
If the patient is unable to handle change in one or two surface characteristics, this indicates difficulty with near transfer.[60]* An inability to handle a change of three to six surface characteristics indicates difficulty with intermediate transfer.

TEST 2: DYNAMIC INTERACTIONAL ASSESSMENT[28,63]

Description:
D.I.A. is not one specific test, but rather a qualitative, process-oriented evaluation. The components of the evaluation are an awareness assessment, strategy investigation and task grading and rsponse to cuing.

Scoring:
The strategies the patient utilizes in a given task are identified (through observation and probing questions). Cues and tasks are altered if the patient has difficulty. The therapist identifies how many task characteristics can be changed before performance breaks down. The patient's ability for near, intermediate and for transfer are evaluated. The types of cuing and task alteration that facilitate patient performance are also recorded. Strategy use is evaluated and recorded in a variety of environments (multicontext).

Treatment of Generalization and Transfer
Utilizing a Remedial Approach:*

1. Strategies can be taught to the patient, however, that does not guarantee he will use them.[64] The therapist must provide opportunities and different situations where the patient may apply them.
2. Generalization requires that the patient recognize that the new situation is similar to an old one.[63]

---

*The remedial approach should only be used if the patient has demonstrated at least near transfer ability.

3. Research has shown "…strategies learned in therapy will generalize to the real world to the extent that the client learns mental organizations that transfer intact…"[11]

4. If the goal is a transferable skill, for example, to use when the patient returns to work, create a simulated work environment and visit the patient's employer. Ensure the patient that he has the necessary skills by performing the targeted job tasks.[11]

5. The skills required to perform complex tasks do not transfer well; successful performance requires practice under conditions that closely match the intended context.[65] Use near transfer tasks for complex skills.

Utilizing an Adaptive Approach:

1. Apply concepts from Dynamic Interactional Theory as follows:

a. Target the processing strategies or behaviors you want to teach the patient in a variety of different tasks.[11,28]

b. Begin with near transfer tasks and use the same strategies in tasks that progressively differ in surface characteristics.[28]

c. Provide multicontext training and teach the patient the variety of conditions to which the strategy can be applied.[28]

d. Increase task complexity when the patient has demonstrated that he can use the strategy effectively in a variety of different situations.[28]

2. Identify the patient's potential placements and plan treatment so that the context doesn't require the patient to reorganize or unlearn anything. For example, placement of hygiene and dressing items should be consistent every day. The patient's kitchen and job site station should also remain consistent. Provide environmental adaptations and cuing through written instructions to compensate for patient's impaired generalization ability.

3. Utilize external aids such as audiotaped instructions, signs, etc., to assist patient in daily occupational performance tasks.

4. Educate the patient and his family as to the generalization and/or transfer deficit and the need for consistent routines and environmental setup.

References

1. Benedict RHB. The effectiveness of cognitive remediation strategies for victims of traumatic head-injury: A review of the literature. *Clinical Psych Review.* 1989;9:605-626.

2. Parente R. Executive skills training. In: Parente R, Herrmann D. (eds.) *Retraining Cognition: Techniques and Application.* Aspen Publications, Gaithersburg, MD (scheduled for publication 1996).

3. Glosser G, Goodglass H. Disorders in executive control functions among aphasic and other brain-damaged patients. *J Clin and Exper Psych.* 1990;12(4):485-501.

4. Levine SP, Horstmann HM, Kirsch NL. Performance considerations for people with cognitive impairment in accessing assistive technologies. *J Head Trauma Rehabil.* 1992;7(3):46-58.

5. Stuss DT. Biological and psychological development of executive functions. *Brain and Cogn.* 1992;20:8-23.

6. Ylvisaker M, Szekeres SF. Metacognitive and executive impairments in head-injured children and adults. *Top Lang Disord.* 1989;9(2):34-49.

7. Zemke R. Task skills, problem solving, and social interaction. In: Royeen CB (ed.). AOTA Self Study Series: *Cognitive Rehabilitation.* American Occupational Therapy Association, Inc.; 1994.

8. Case R. The role of the frontal lobes in the regulation of cognitive development. *Brain and Cogn.* 1992;20:51-73.

9. Cook EA, Thigpen R. Identification and management of cognitive and perceptual deficits in the rehabilitation patient. *Rehabilitation Nursing.* Sept/Oct 1993;18(5):3110-3113.

10. Lezak M. *Neuropsychological Assessment.* New York, Oxford University Press; 1983.

11. Parente R. Effect of monetary incentives on performance after traumatic brain injury. *Neuro Rehabil.* 1994;4(3):198-203.

12. Barco P, Grosson B, Bolesta MM, Werts D, Stout R. Training awareness and compensation in postacute head injury rehabilitation. In: Kreutzer JS, Wehman PH (eds.) *Cognitive Rehabilitation For Persons with Traumatic Brain Injury: A Functional Approach.* Baltimore, Paul H. Brooks Publishing Co.; 1991.

13. Anderson SW, Tranel D. Awareness of disease states following cerebral infarction, dementia, and head trauma: Standardized assessment. *The Clinical Neuropsychologist.* 1989;3(4):327-339.

14. Doehring DG, Reitan RM, Klove H. Changes in patterns of intelligence test performance associated wih homonymous visual field defects. *J Nerv Ment Dis.* 1961;132:227-233.

15. Gasquoine PG, Gibbons TA. Lack of awareness of impairment in institutionalized, severely and chronically disabled survivors of traumatic brain injury: A preliminary investigation. *J Head Trauma Rehabil.* 1994;9(4):16-24.

16. Prigatano GP, Altman IM, O'Brien KP. Behavioral limitations that traumatic-brain-injured patients tend to underestimate. *Clinical Neuropsychologist.* 1990;4(2):163-176.

17. Prigatano GP. Disturbances of self-awareness of deficit after traumatic brain injury. In: Prigatano GP, Schacter DL (eds.). *Awareness of Deficit After Brain Injury.* New York, Oxford University Press; 1991.

18. Schacter DL, Prigatano GP. Forms of unawareness. In: Prigatano GP, Schacter DL (eds.). *Awareness of Deficit After Injury.* New York, Oxford University Press; 1991.

19. Hansen CS. Traumatic brain injury. In: Van Deusen J (ed.). *Body Image and Perceptual Dysfunction in Adults.* Philadelphia, WB Saunders; 1993.

20. McGlynn SM. Behavioral approaches to neuropsychological rehabilitation. *Psychological Bulletin.* 1990;108(3):420-441.

21. Ayres AJ. *Southern California Sensory Integration Tests.* Los Angeles, Western Psychological Services; 1972.

22. Namerow NS. Cognitive and behavioral aspects of brain-injury rehabilitation. *Neurologic Rehab.* Nov 1987;5(4):569-583.

23. Bruce MAG. Cognitive rehabilitation: Intelligence, insight, and knowledge. In: Royeen CB (ed.). AOTA Self Study Series: *Cognitive Rehabilitation.* American Occupational Therapy Association, Inc.; 1994.

24. Harrington DO. *The Visual Fields* (4th edition). St. Louis, CV Mosby Co.; 1976.

25. Lewinsohn PM, Zieler RE, Lilet J, Eyeberg S, Nielson G. Short-term memory. *J Compar Physiol Psychol.* 1972;1072(81):248-255.

26. Cohen RF, Mapou RL. Neuropsychological assessment for treatment planning: A hypothesis-testing approach. *J Head Trauma Rehabil.* 1988;3(1):12-23.

27. Grafman J, Kampen D, Rosenberg J, Salazar AM, Boller F. The progressive breakdown of number processing and calculation ability: A case study. *Cortex.* 1989;25:121-133.

28. Toglia JP. Attention and memory. AOTA Self Study Series: *Cognitive Rehabilitation.* The American Occupational Therapy Association; 1994.

29. Craine JF. The retraining of frontal lobe dysfunction. In: Trexler LE (ed.). *Cognitive Rehabilitation: Conceptualization and Invervention.* New York, Plenum Press; 1982.

30. Craine JF, Gudeman HE. *The Rehabilitation of Brain Functions: Principles, Procedures and Techniques of Neurotraining.* Springfield, IL, Charles C. Thomas Pub.; 1981.

31. Rahmani L. The intellectual rehabilitation of brain-damaged patients. *Clin Neuropsychol.* 1982;4:44-45.

32. Cicerone KD, Wood J. Planning disorder after closed head injury: A case study. *Arch Phys Med Rehabil.* 1987;68:111-113.

33. Fetherlin JM, Kurland L. Self-instruction: A compensatory strategy to increase functional independence with brain-injured adults. *Occup Ther Pract.* 1989;1(1):75-78.

34. Bourne LE, Dominowski RL, Loftus EF. *Cognitive Processes.* Englewood Cliffs, NJ, Prentice-Hall, Inc.; 1979.

35. Christenson AL. *Luria's Neuropsychological Investigation.* New York, Spectrum Publications; 1975.

36. Duchek J. Cognitive dimensions of performance. In: Christiansen C, Baum C (eds). *Occupational Therapy: Overcoming Human Performance Deficits.* Thorofare, NJ, SLACK Inc.; 1991.

37. Patterson KE, Baddeley AD. When face recognition fails. *J Exp Psychol Hum Learn Mem.* 1977;3:406-417.

38. Goldstein FC, Levin H. Disorders of reasoning and problem solving ability. In: Meir MJ, Benton AL, Diller L. (eds). *Neuropsychological Rehabilitation.* New York, Guilford University Press; 1987.

39. Meltzer M. Poor memory: A case report. *J Clin Psychol.* 1983;39(1):3-10.

40. Rabbit P. Changes in problem solving ability in old age. In: Birren J, Schaie K (eds.). *Handbook of Psychology of Aging.* New York, Von Nostrand Reinhold Co.; 1977.

41. Hoyer W, Rebok G, Svold S. Effects of varying irrelevant information on adult age differences in problm solving. *J Gerontol.* 1979;34(4):553-560.

42. Layton B. Perceptual noise and aging. *Psychol Bull.* 1975;82:875-883.

43. Schonfield D. Translations in gerontology—from lab to life: Utilizing information. *Am Psychol.* 1974;29:796-901.

44. Adamovich BLB. Cognition, language, attention and information processing following closed head injury. In: Kreutzer JS, Wehman PH (eds) *Cognitive Rehabilitation For Persons with Traumatic Brain Injury: A Functional Approach.* Baltimore, Paul H. Brooks Publishing Co.; 1991.

45. Ben-Yishay Y, Diller L. Cognitive remediation. In: Griffith E, Bond M, Miller J. (eds). *Rehabilitation of the Head Injured Adult.* Philadelphia, FA Davis; 1983b.

46. Bolger J. Cognitive retraining: A developmental approach. *Clin Neuropsychol.* 1982;4:55-70.

47. Prigatano GP. *Neuropsychological Rehabilitation After Brain Injury.* Baltimore, Johns Hopkins University Press; 1986.

48. Okkema, K. *Cognition and Perception in the Stroke Patient.* Gaithersburg, Aspen Publishers; 1993.

49. Zoltan B. Visual, visual perceptual and perceptual-motor deficits in brain injured adults: Evaluation, treatment and functional implications. In: Kraft GH, Berrol S (eds). *Physical Medicine and Rehabilitation Clinics of North America.* Philadelphia, WB Saunders Co.; 1992.

50. VonCramon DY, Matthes-VonCramon G, Mai N. The influence of a cognitive remediation programme on associated behavioural disturbances in patients with frontal lobe dysfunction. In: VonSteinbuchel N, VonCramon DY, Poppel E (eds.). *Neuropyschological Rehabilitation.* Berlin, Springer-Verlag; 1992.

51. Dougherty PM, Radomski MV. *A Dynamic Assessment Approach for Adults with Brain Injury: The Cognitive Rehabilitation Workbook.* Gaithersburg, MD, Aspen Publishers; 1993.

52. Arenberg D, Robertson-Tchabo E. Learning and aging. In: Birren J, Schaie K (eds): *Handbook of the Psychology of Aging.* New York, Von Nostrand Reinhold Co.; 1977.

53. Grafman J. Plans, actions, and mental sets: Managerial knowledge units in the frontal lobes. In: Perecman E (ed.). *Integrating Theory and Practice in Clinical Neuropsychology.* Hillsdale, NJ, Lawrence Erlbaum Assoc.; 1989.

54. Parker RS. *Traumatic Brain Injury and Neuropsychological Impairment.* New York, Springer-Verlag; 1990.

55. VanZomeren AH, Fasotti L. Impairments of attention in brain-damaged patients. In: VonSteinbuchel N, VonCramon DY, Poppel E (eds.). *Neuropsychological Rehabilitation.* Berlin, Springer-Verlag; 1992.

56. Malec J. Training the brain-injured client in behavioral self-management skills. In: Edelstein BA, Couture ET (eds.). *Behavioral Assessment and Rehabilitation of the Traumatically Brain-Damaged.* New York, Plenum Press; 1984.

57. Ben-Yishay Y, Diller L. Cognitive remediation in traumatic brain injury: Update and issues. *Arch Phys Med Rehabil.* 1993;74:204-213.

58. Goldstein G. Comprehensive neuropsychological assessment batteries. In: Goldstein G, Hersen M (eds.). *Handbook of Psychological Assessment.* New York, Pergamon Press; 1984.

59. Ben-Yishay Y, et al. *Working Approaches to Remediation of Cognitive Deficits in Brain-damaged Persons. Rehabilitation Monograph 62.* New York, New York University Medical Center, May 1981.

60. Neistadt ME. Assessing learning capabilities during cognitive and perceptual evaluations for adults with traumatic brain injury. *Occup Ther in Health Care.* 1995;9(1):3-16.

61. Ullman M. Disorder of body image after stroke. *Am J Nurs.* 1964;64:89-91.

62. Woolcock WW. Generalization Strategies. In: Wehman P, Kreutzer JS (eds). *Vocational Rehabilitation for Persons with Traumatic Head Injury.* Rockville, MD, Aspen Publishers; 1990.

63. Toglia JP. Generalization of treatment: A multicontextual approach to cognitive perceptual impairment in the brain injured adult. *Amer J Occup Ther.* 1991;45(6):505-516.

64. Wilson B. Coping strategies for memory dysfunction. In: Perecman E (ed.). *Integrating Theory and Practice in Clinical Neuropsychology.* Hillsdale, NJ, Lawrence Erlbaum Assoc; 1989.

65. Vezzetti D. Capacity, content, control: A model for analyzing the cognitive demands of activity. *Occup Ther Pract.* 1989;1(1):9-17.

CHAPTER 10

Acalculia

The ability to perform calculations is crucial to many areas of occupational performance. The skill is used for everything from reading price tags to using the phone to addressing letters and writing checks.[1] Apart from language, calculation is perhaps the only culturally determined semantic system that the majority of the population is expected to acquire and master.[2] Impairment in number processing and calculations frequently accompanies focal and diffuse brain damage.[3]

In order to understand and interpret any problems the patient may have with calculations, it is important to understand the theoretical underlying mechanisms required for successful performance. It is generally assumed that the cognitive numerical processing mechanisms include numeral comprehension, numeral production and cognitive processes specific to arithmetic.[4] It includes components of comprehension of operation symbols (ie, +) and words (plus), retrieval of arithmetic facts and execution of calculation procedures.[4,5]

The number processing system is generally distinguished from the calculation system. The number processing system includes the number comprehension and number production subsystems.[5] The calculation system, on the other hand, includes the comprehension of operation symbols, the retrieval of arithmetic facts, and the execution of arithmetic procedures.[1,4-6] Within each of these subsystems, a further distinction is made between components for processing Arabic number (ie, numbers in digit form such as 362) and components for processing verbal numbers.[1]

The number comprehension subsystem translates Arabic or verbal number inputs into internal semantic representations for use in subsequent cognitive processing.[1] Within the Arabic and verbal number comprehension components, a distinction is made between lexical and syntactic processing. Lexical processing is the comprehension of the individual elements in a number. For example, the digit 3 or the word three. Syntactic processing involves the analysis of the relations among elements. This skill refers to word order or the ability to produce an internal representation of the number as a whole.[1]

As previously described, number production components serve to translate internal semantic representations of numbers into sequences of digit or word representations for output.[1,6] Performing calculations requires the three elements of cognitive processes for number com-

Dyscalculia Battery: Number-Processing Section*

	Item	Correct Response
Magnitude Comparison Tasks		
Arabic Numbers	108	
		Point to '150'
	150	
Spoken verbal numbers	☐ 'fifty'	
		Point to square representing 'fifty'
	☐ 'fifteen'	
Written verbal numbers	eleven thousand eighteen	
		Point to 'eleven thousand eighteen'
	three hundred eighty-five	
Transcoding Tasks		
Arabic to spoken verbal numbers	190	'one hundred ninety'
Spoken verbal to written verbal numbers	'nineteen'	nineteen
Spoken verbal to Arabic numbers	'four thousand fifty-seven'	4,057
Arabic to written verbal numbers	5	five
Written verbal to spoken verbal numbers	ninety-two	'ninety-two'
Written verbal to Arabic numbers	three thousand twenty-four	3,024

Figure 10-1. Examples of test items from the number-processing section of the dyscalculia test battery.[1] Reproduced with permission from Oxford University Press, 198 Madison Ave, New York, NY.

prehension and production and cognitive processes that are specific to calculation procedures. These processes include comprehension of operation symbols or words, retrieval of number facts and execution of the procedures themselves. Retrieval of number facts is central to almost any form of arithmetic problem solving.[6]

The number processing and calculation system model is summarized in Figure 10-1 and Figure 10-2. Although the number processing and calculation system model is generally accepted, some theorists believe it to be somewhat oversimplified.[7] An alternative theory of encoding complex has been proposed. These theorists hypothesize that excitatory and inhibitory associative processes contribute collectively to the performance of numerical tasks. Rather than assuming that brain damage would selectively impair comprehension, calculation or production, this model suggests that partial dysfunction might by associated with selective damage to inhibitory processes.[7] A non-modular system, in which multiple numerical codes activate one another in the course of numeral processing and arithmetic tasks, is envisioned.[4] These numerical codes are assumed to be interconnected in an associative network.

Whether or not one accepts a modular or encoding complex model of number processing

Dyscalculia Battery: Calculation Section*

Operation Symbol and Word Comprehension Tasks	Item	Correct Response
Operation symbol comprehension	subtraction 6 + 2 6 X 2 6 • 2	Point to '6 • 2'
Operation word comprehension	addition 'nine times six'	'No'
Written Arithmetic Tasks		
Addition	752 +978	752 +978 1730
Subtraction	86 -37	86 -37 49
Multiplication	30 x 84	30 x 84 120 2400 2520
Oral Arithmetic Tasks		
Addition	'five plus eight'	'thirteen'
Subtraction	'seventeen minus nine'	'eight'
Multiplication	'six times three'	'eighteen'

Figure 10-2. Examples of test items from the calculation section of the dyscalculia test battery.[1] Reproduced with permission from Oxford University Press, 198 Madison Ave, New York, NY.

and calculations is less crucial than how the specific skills are manifest clinically. Acalculia usually occurs with a number of other deficits, such as aphasia or as part of Gerstmanns syndrome.[8] It can, however, be seen as a primary deficit involving all four arithmetic operations.[5] One study has also described a patient who exhibited acalculia for addition, subtraction and division, but had intact multiplication.[5] This patient also had intact ability to distinguish math signs. These results point to the possibility of different processing systems which are responsible for each of the basic arithmetic operations.

Tohgi et al[9] support these findings in a description of a patient with a left frontal lobe infarct. The patient was able to add and subtract numbers, but could not multiply or divide. The deficit was attributed to a difficulty in retrieving facts from the multiplication tables and the calculation procedures themselves.

Corbett et al,[10] describe still another clinical picture related to acalculia. A 60-year-old male with a subcortical infarct had difficulties in numerical syntax, a loss of ability to manipulate math concepts and impaired working memory. This study is one of several which have demonstrated that localization for number processing and calculations is not limited to cortical structures.[11]

Sokol et al[12] describe a T.B.I. patient with impaired retrieval of arithmetic facts but intact abilities in execution of calculation procedures. These authors point to two separate functionally distinct components in the cognitive calculation system.

Rosselli and Ardila[13] studied 41 patients with left hemisphere damage and 21 patients with right hemisphere damage. All groups presented difficulties with calculations tasks. Left hemisphere patients showed significantly higher number of errors in reading numbers and arithmetic signs, counting backwards, and performing successive operations. These patients however, showed a better comprehension of written numbers. Lucchelli and DeRenzi[14] also describe a patient with good comprehension of operation symbols, but impaired retrieval of math facts and execution of calculation procedures.

Takayama et al[15] describe patients who could read, repeat and accurately verbalize numbers; had normal counting ability; understood the basic processes of calculation and showed little difficulty in the retrieval of table values. Their errors were made in the process where a number of steps were carried out simultaneously. These steps included retrieval of the number fact or table value, appropriate spatial alignment of the digits, appropriate procedural access and retention and appropriate use of any integers remaining from the previous product.[15] These authors concluded that a working memory deficit could have a strong effect on multi-digit arithmetic problems, and that the left parietal lobe may be a specialized area for working memory for calculation.[15]

The previously described theoretical models and supporting research studies indicate that acalculia can be manifest in a number of different ways. The deficit can have broad implications relating to occupational performance and therefore warrants a complete evaluation.

Evaluation of Acalculia

TEST 1: DYSCALCULIA BATTERY[1]

Description:
This test battery has items representing both the number processing system and calculations system. Within each of these major sections are items covering all the component skills. Please refer to Figure 10-1 and Figure 10-2 for examples of test items.

TEST 2: FUNCTIONAL CALCULATIONS EVALUATION

Description:
An evaluation can be developed that contains test items for recognition of numbers, simple mathematical operations and complex mathematical operations, including concepts associated with these operations.[16,17] Test items that are functionally oriented should be incorporated into the evaluation, eg, coin recognition, calculating change, check writing or budgeting.

Scoring:
Nonstandardized. The clinician measures the patient's level of performance on each category of tasks described.
To improve validity, rule out poor visual attentiveness and oculomotor skills, decreased attention, problem solving, mental inflexibility and aphasia as causes of poor performance.

Treatment for Acalculia

Utilizing a Remedial Approach:

1. Identify which aspect or aspects of the number processing or calculations system are impaired. Ask the patient to perform repetitive related tasks beginning with one-step operations and progressing to multiple step operations as the patient improves.
2. Utilize computer retraining with software that has been designed for the specific remediation of number processing and calculations skills.

Utilizing an Adaptive Approach:

1. Identify how the patient's acalculia is affecting function and provide environmental adaptations as needed. For example, if the patient is unable to balance his or her checkbook, checkbook calculators can be utilized. If using a telephone is a problem, then a telephone with memory can assist. Basic calculators may also be utilized for number operations required in the school, home or work setting.

References

1. Macaruso P, Harley W, McCloskey M. Assessment of acquired dyscalculia. In: Margolin DM (ed.). *Cognitive Neuropsychology in Clinical Practice.* New York: Oxford University Press; 1992:405-434.
2. Spiers PA. Acalculia revisited: current issues. In: Deloche G, Seron X, eds. *Mathematical Disabilities: A Cognitive Neuropsychological Perspective.* Hillsdale, NJ: Lawrence Erlbaum Assoc. Pubs.; 1987.
3. Benson DF. Disorders of visual gnosis. In: Brown JW, ed. *Neuropsychology of Visual Perception.* Hillsdale, NJ: Lawrence Erlbaum Assoc.; 1989.
4. McCloskey M. Cognitive mechanisms in numerical processing: evidence from acquired dyscalculia. *Cognition.* 1992;44:107-157.
5. Lample Y, Eshel Y, Gilad R, Sarova-Pinhas I. Selective acalculia with sparing of the subtraction process in a patient with left parietotemporal hemorrhage. *Neurology.* Sept 1994;44:1759-1761.
6. McCloskey M, Harley W, Sokol SM. Models of arithmetic fact retrieval: an evaluation in light of findings from normal and brain-damaged subjects. *J Exp Psych Learning Mem Cogn.* 1991;17(3):377-397.
7. Clark JM, Campbell JID. Integrated versus modular theories of number skills and acalculia. *Brain and Cogn.* 1991;17:204-239.
8. Grafman J, Kampen D, Rosenberg J, Salazar AM, Boller F. The progressive breakdown of number processing and calculation ability: a case study. *Cortex.* 1989;25:121-133.
9. Tohgi H, Saitoh K, Takahashi S, et al. Agraphia and acalculia after a left prefrontal (F1, F2) infarction. *J Neurol Neurosurg Psychiatry.* 1995;58:629-632.
10. Corbett AJ, McCusker EA, Davidson OR. Acalculia following a dominant-hemisphere subcortical infarct. *Arch Neurol.* Sept 1986:43:964-966.

11. Kahn HJ, Whitaker HA. Acalculia: An historical review of localization. *Brain and Cogn.* 1991;17:102-1151.

12. Sokol SM, McCloskey M, Cohen NJ, Aliminosa D. Cognitive representations and processes in arithmetic: Inferences from the performance of brain-damaged subjects. *J Exp Psych Learning Mem Cogn.* 1991;17(3):355-376.

13. Rosselli M, Ardila A. Alculation deficits in patients with right and left hemisphere damage. *Neuropsychologia.* 1989;27(5):607-617.

14. Lucchelli F, DeRenzi E. Primary dyscalculia after a medical frontal lesion of the left hemisphere. *J Neurol Neurosurg Psychiatry.* 1993;56:304-307.

15. Takayama Y, Sugishita M, Akiguchi I, Kimura J. Isolated acalculia due to left parietal lesion. *Arch Neurol.* Mar 1994;1:286-291.

16. Lezak M. *Neuropsychological Assessment.* New York: Oxford University Press; 1983.

17. Luria AR. *Higher Cortical Functions in Man.* 2nd ed. New York: Basic Books, Inc.; 1980.

CHAPTER 11

Factors that Influence the Patient's Vision, Perception and Cognition

Many areas of skill have an influence on the patient's vision, perception or cognition. For example, aphasia, sensory loss, and visual and perceptual deficits can all complicate or interfere with the patient's cognitive abilities. Detailed information about these areas has been presented elsewhere in this book. In addition to these areas, age and environment can influence the patient's cognitive, perceptual and visual skills. The effects of age and environment on cognition are described in this chapter.

The Relationship of Age to Visual, Perceptual and Cognitive Evaluation and Treatment

The incidence of C.V.A. escalates rapidly with advancing age, from 3.3 per 100,000 persons under 35 to 1800 or more in those 85 years old or older.[1] One study reports that, of 578 patients who had sustained C.V.A.'s, 76.5 percent were between the ages of 60 and 99 years.[2] A similar study reports that 81 percent of the population were between 65 and 74 years of age and 92.5 percent were between 75 and 84 years.[1]

Despite research and clinical evidence that the majority of the patients who sustain a C.V.A. are elderly, functional, neurological changes that occur as the result of normal aging are rarely taken into account during visual, perceptual and cognitive evaluation and treatment. The following section is an attempt to acquaint the reader with the major changes related to the normal aging process that may affect visual, perceptual and cognitive functioning.

Sensory Loss

Vision

Visual acuity and adaptability decline with age.[3-6] Decreased depth perception and peri-

Table 11-1. Changes in the Visual System Associated with Age

Structural Component	Age Related Change	Functional Implications
Cornea	1. Appearance change	Loss of luster, limited amount of fluid bathing the cornea
	2. Accumulation of lipids	Increased astigmatism with increased blurred vision (independent of near or farsightedness)
Iris	Decreased permeability	May contribute to glaucoma
Ciliary Muscle	Atrophy of muscle	Decreased mobility of the lens which causes decreased muscle effectiveness
Pupil	1. Decreased pupil size	Restricted amount of light reaching retina; difficulty in seeing dark objects or objects in dim light
	2. Decreased pupillary reflex	Decreased dark adaptation and recovery from glare
Lens	1. Lens growth	Decreased accommodative ability
	2. Decreased refractive index of lenses	Uneven refracture properties, which can result in double vision in one eye
	3. Yellowing	Reduces amount of light reaching retina and changes light composition; alters color vision
Vitreous	Contracts	May separate from retina (the retina itself may also detach)

pheral vision may also occur.[7] Changes occur in the cornea, pupil, iris, lens, vitreous, and ciliary muscles of the eyes.[3,5,7,8] These changes are summarized in Table 11-1.

Audition

Hearing losses caused by aging are always bilateral and usually symmetrical.[9] Age-related changes might include decreased inner ear function, thickening of the tympanic membrane, loss of elasticity of the ossicular chain, and atrophy of the cochlea or organ or Corti.[7,9] As a result of the structural changes of the auditory system, any or all of the following functional changes might occur:

1. High frequency loss
2. All frequency loss
3. Neural problems that result in decreased speech comprehension and discrimination
4. Problems in determining the source of a sound
5. Distortion of environmental sound
6. Difficulty hearing in the presence of background noise
7. Impaired intellectual functioning.

Remaining Sensory Systems

Research has indicated that in at least a portion of the elderly population, there is a reduced sensitivity to taste, smell, touch, vibration, temperature, kinesthesia, and pain.[3,10]

Autonomic Nervous System

Age-related changes in the hypothalamus have been observed and seem to result in decreased maintenance of homeostasis.[11,12] Age-related changes occur in the metabolism and regulatory mechanisms of an organism. Aging is "characterized by a progressive decrease in the intensity of adaptive processes."[13] It is believed that with aging, autonomic nervous system changes take place throughout all aspects of the system. These changes lead to shifts in the reflectory regulation of inner organs, a decrease in the organism's adaptive capacities, a decrease in the reliability of homeostatic regulatory mechanisms, an easier disruption of regulatory mechanisms, and the development of disorders in old age.[12]

Perception

In view of the close relationship between vision and perception, it can be expected that age-related visual changes will influence perceptual abilities in the elderly. For example, the decreased accommodative power and poor lens transmissiveness previously described can in turn affect distance vision, sensitivity to glare, and depth and color perception.[8] Losses in acuity and distance perception,[8] visual closure, or part-whole perception may also be deficient. The elderly patient may exhibit decreased visual discrimination, figure-ground, visual memory and spatial relations.[14] The quality of stereopsis depends on brightness and contrast. Therefore, any age-related process that reduces retinal illumination would impair binocular depth perception.[8] Decreased pattern recognition and poor attentional processing during visual search have also been documented.[15-17]

In addition to distance, depth, and color perception, the elderly's visual fields may be altered. This age-related change involves the retina and the nervous system in general. Age-related circulatory changes can cause a metabolic change in the retina, which in turn is reflected by changes in the size of the visual field.[8]

Cognition

Research has indicated that decreased brain weight and volume and a decrease in the cells of the cerebral cortex occur with age.[18,19] Since the cerebral cortex is intricately involved with higher intellectual functioning, cognitive and behavioral changes might be expected with age. Nearly all aspects of human performance are guided by cognition.[20] The following is an overview of documented age-related cognitive impairments.

The documentation of decreased memory of one type of another in the elderly is abundant.[21-32] Some authors believe that age-related memory loss is primarily a storage and retrieval problem. Others believe that nonverbal memory is a particular problem for the elderly, and that they will benefit from the use of verbal cues to improve their performance.[29,31] Craik, Byrd and Swanson[24] believe age-related deficits in memory appear to be related to cognitive tasks that require a greater amount of effort for processing than automatic processing. Age-related memory loss has also been attributed to the inefficient use of learning strategies.[21,33] For example, the elderly do not use repetition, visual imagery, verbal mediation, association encoding, mnemonics, or organization strategies as often or as effectively as younger individuals.[21,33,34] Inefficient use of all or any of these strategies means that the retrieval cues are minimal.[21] Retrieval deficits in the elderly in association with new information do not appear to generalize to very old memory. In addition, recent research has indicated that any changes with aging in either the capacity or duration of iconic memory are slight if they exist at all.[15] No major changes in echoic memory were noted.[15]

Decreased spatial memory has also been documented in the elderly.[26] Age differences in face recognition memory are also apparent by the fifth decade.[25] This difference becomes especially pronounced by the seventh decade.[25] Additional age-related deficits include a decreased ability to acquire knowledge about a novel environment, and decreased bilateral coordination.[24]

A generalized slowing of cognitive processes and reaction time in the elderly has also been documented.[35] There is diminished ability for abstract and complex conceptualization, and poor mental flexibility.[3,33] These deficits, along with decreased memory, can cause difficulty in adapting to new situations, solving novel problems, and changing from one mental set to another.[3,33] There is indeed documentation of poor problem solving ability among the elderly.[3,36-38]

Implications for Evaluation

Some of the age-related deficits described in this section may or may not be present in a given individual. It is vital for the occupational therapist to obtain a clear picture of the C.V.A. patient's premorbid status prior to visual, perceptual or cognitive evaluation and treatment. Vision should be evaluated prior to testing, and measures that involve small visual stimuli should be avoided if possible. Responses that require fine color discrimination, especially in the blue spectrum, may be invalid.[39] One should use color contrasts, an increased amount of light, and clean prescription glasses when indicated. Determine the patient's hearing acuity. Evaluate the effects of modifying your voice, identify the best position to sit or stand to reinforce what is said, and make sure that the patient's hearing aid is clean.[7] Consult vision and hearing experts when there is a question.

Always remember that for the elderly, testing is often a threatening experience. The fear of testing may in fact limit their risk taking and inhibit their response. Consider the environment when testing: the elderly are more easily distracted by irrelevant stimuli than younger individuals.[40]

Finally, consider fatigue in testing.[21,33] Mental fatigue at any age can cause various sensory and perceptual changes, slowed and disorganized performance, and perhaps short-term memory impairment.[40]

Implications in Treatment

The areas to consider for evaluation are also applicable to treatment. In addition, the therapist should limit redundant and extraneous information and treat in a non-distracting environment.[21,31] Repetition and practice are indicated because the elderly (along with the young) can benefit from this.[21] For example, research has shown that the elderly, like the young, have the capability of improving their skill in divided attention through practice.[41] Intensive and extensive mnemonics training can also help the elderly.[32] Formal training in mnemonics has increased the learning proficiency of some elderly adults.[32] The extent of benefit, however, depends on the extent of training.

Allow sufficient time for the patient to respond and utilize cues that will most benefit the patient, eg, verbal, visual, touch, or movement in addition to practice and cuing. The elderly patient who has sustained a C.V.A. can benefit from controlled sensory stimulation and sensory integrative techniques.[42] These treatment approaches are covered in detail in Chapter 1.

References

1. Robins M, Baum H. Incidence, Part II. *Stroke.* 1981;12(2):45-58.
2. Moskowitz E, Lightbody EEH, Freitag NS. Long-term follow-up of the post stroke patient. *Arch Phys Med Rehab.* 1972;53:167-172.
3. Filskov S, Boll T. *Handbook of Clinical Neuropsychology.* New York: John Wiley & Sons, Inc.; 1981.
4. Hoyer WJ, Rybash JM. Age and visual field differences in computing visual-spatial relations. *Psych & Aging.* 1992;7(3):339-342.
5. Podolsky S, Schachar R. Clinical manifestations of diabetic retinopathy and other diseases of the eye in the elderly. In: Ordy JM, Bizzee KR, eds. *Aging. Vol. 10. Sensory Systems and Communication in the Elderly.* New York: Raven Press; 1979.
6. Vaughan WJ, Smitz P, Fatt I. The human lens—a model system for the study of aging. In: Ordy JM, Bizzee KR, eds. *Aging. Vol. 10. Sensory Systems and Communication in the Elderly.* New York: Raven Press; 1979.
7. Buseck S, Sheilds E. Aging: sensory losses. Available from American Journal of Nursing Co., Educational Services Division, 555 W. 57th Street, New York, New York. (Study guide and videotape.)
8. Fozard J, Wolf E, Bell B, McFarland R, Podolsky S. Visual perception and communication. In: Birren J, Schaie K, eds. *Handbook of Psychology of Aging.* New York: Van Nostrand Reinhold Co.; 1977.
9. Pickett JM, Bergman M, Levitt H. Aging and speech understanding. In: Ordy JM, Bizzee KR, eds. *Aging. Vol. 10. Sensory Systems and Communication in the Elderly.* New York: Raven Press; 1979.
10. Jackson OL. Brain function, aging, and dementia, In: Umphred DA, ed. *Neurological Rehabilitation.* 2nd ed. St. Louis: C.V. Mosby Co.; 1990.
11. Diamond MC. The aging brain: some enlightening and optimistic results. *Am Scient.* 1978;66:66-71.
12. Frolkis V. Aging of the autonomic nervous system. In: Birren J, Schaie K, eds. *Handbook of the Psychology of Aging.* New York: Van Nostrand Reinhold Co.; 1977.
13. Drachman D, Leavitt J. Memory impairment in the aged: storage vs. retrieval deficit. *J Exp Psychol.* 1972;93(2):302-308.
14. Su CY, Chien TH, Cheng KF, Lin TY. Performance of older adults with and without cerebrovascular accident on the test of visual perceptual skills. *Am J Occup Ther.* 1995;49(6):491-499.
15. Kausler DH. *Learning and Memory in Normal Aging.* San Diego: Academic Press; 1994.
16. Madden DJ. Adult age differences in the time course of visual attention. *Journal of Gerontology.* 1990;45,9-16.

17. Russo R, Parkin AJ. Age differences in implicit memory, more apparent than real. *Memory and Cognition.* 1993;21:73-80.
18. Bondareff W. The neural basis of aging. In: Birren J, Schaie K, eds. *Handbook of the Psychology of Aging.* New York: Van Nostrand Reinhold Co.; 1977.
19. Brody H, Vijayashankar N. Anatomical changes in the nervous system. In: Finch CE, Hayfbeck L, eds. *Handbook of the Biology of Aging.* New York: Van Nostrand Reinhold Co.; 1977.
20. Duchek J. Cognitive dimensions of performance. In: Christiansen C, Baum C, eds. *Occupational Therapy: Overcoming Human Performance Deficits.* Thorofare, NJ: SLACK Inc.; 1991.
21. Arenberg D, Robertson-Tchabo E. Learning and aging. In: Birren J, Schaie K, eds. *Handbook of the Psychology of Aging.* New York: Van Nostrand Reinhold Co.; 1977; 421-449.
22. Baum B, Hall K. Relationship between constructional praxis and dressing in the head injured adult. *Am J Occup Ther.* 1981;35(7):438-442.
23. Birren J, Renner V. Research on the psychology of aging: principles and experimentation. In: Birren J, Schaie K, eds. *Handbook of the Psychology of Aging.* New York: Van Nostrand Reinhold Co.; 1977.
24. Craik FIM, Byrd M, Swanson JL. Patterns of memory loss in three elderly samples. *Psychology and Aging.* 1987;2:79-86.
25. Crook TH, Larrabee GJ. Changes in facial recognition memory across the adult lifespan. *The Journal of Gerentology: Psychological Sciences.* 1992;47:138-141.
26. Denneg NW, Dew JR, Kihlstrom JF. An adult developmental study of the encoding of spatial location., *Experimental Aging Research.* 1992;18:25-32.
27. Kahn RL, Zarit SH, Hilbert NM, Neiderehe G. Memory complaints and impairment in the aged. *Arch Gen Psychiat.* 1975;32:1569-1573.
28. Kolb B, Wishaw. *I.Q. Fundamentals of Human Neuropsychology.* New York: N.H. Freeman and Co.; 1990.
29. Kramer N, Farbik L. Assessment of intellectual changes in the elderly. In: Raskin A, Jarbik L, eds. *Psychiatric Symptoms and Cognitive Loss in the Elderly.* New York: Hemisphere Pub. Co.; 1979.
30. Riege W, Inman V. Age differences in nonverbal memory tasks. *J Gerontol.* 1979;36(1):51-58.
31. Riege WH, Klane LT, Metter EJ, Hanson WR. Decision speed and bias after unilateral stroke. *Cortex.* 1982;18:345-355.
32. Verhaegen P, Marcoen A, Grossenms L. Improving memory performance in the aged through mneumonic training: a meta-analytic study. *Psychology and Aging.* 1992;7:242-251.
33. Lezak M. *Neuropsychological Assessment.* New York: Oxford University Press; 1983.
34. Brown J. *Aphasia, Apraxia and Agnosia, Clinical and Theoretical Aspects.* Springfield, IL: Charles C Thomas Pub.; 1972.
35. Murrell FH. The effect of extensive practice on age difference in reaction time. *J Gerontol.* 1970;25:268-274.
36. Arenberg D. A longitudinal study of problem solving in adults. *J. Gerontol.* 1974;29:656-658.
37. Rabbit P. Changes in problem solving ability in old age. In: Birren J, Schaie K, (eds.). *Handbook of Psychology of Aging.* New York: Van Nostrand Reinhold Co.; 1977.
38. Young M. Problem-solving performance in two age groups. *J Gerontol.* 1966;21:505-509.
39. Bracy O. Computer based cognitive rehabilitation. *Cognit Rehab.* 1983;1(1):7-8.
40. Crook T. Psychometric assessment in the elderly. In: Raskin A, Javick L, eds. *Psychiatric Symptoms and Cognitive Loss in the Elderly.* New York: Hemisphere Publishing Co.; 1979:207-220.
41. Barron A, Mattila WR. Response slowing of older adults: effects of time limit contingencies on single and dual task performances. *Psychology and Aging.* 1989;4:66-72.
42. Ordy JM, Brizzee KR. Sensory coding: sensation perception, information processing, and sensory-motor integration from maturity to old age. In: Ordy JM, Bizzee KR, eds. *Aging. Vol 10. Sensory Systems and Communication in the Elderly.* New York: Raven Press; 1979.

CHAPTER 12

The Use of Computers in Visual, Perceptual and Cognitive Retraining

The application of computer technology to health care has increased rapidly in recent years. Its use in rehabilitation has become established in the US, Canada, Great Britain, Australia and other developed countries.[1] Probably the most recent use of computers in health care has been in direct patient treatment. Such use can range from prevocational applications, to environmental control, to visual, perceptual, or cognitive retraining.[2-5] Computer programs have been designed and used to assess reaction time, visual scanning, attention, speed of information processing, memory and problem solving.[4,6-9] The concept of using the computer as an adaptive or prosthetic device has also gained popularity.[10-12]

Computer advocates believe computers to be the ultimate in flexibility and readily modifiable.[13] In addition, it is believed computer use saves therapist time, provides an objective measure of performance, and provides immediate feedback to the patient.[14] Computer programs can control stimulus exposure time and level of difficulty, which can be systematically altered to meet the patients individual needs.[14] Small and affordable computers and general availability of hard or fixed discs have expanded the potential for computer use in visual, perceptual or cognitive retraining.[13] In addition to these advances in hardware, new software is available which can modify keyboard use and which is specifically designed for the remediation of cognitive deficits.[2,12,13,15-17]

Despite its apparent advantages and increased use, its effectiveness in visual, perceptual and cognitive retraining remains controversial. Microcomputer based assessment and treatment of visual processing has been examined in a number of empirical studies.[1,8,18] Robertson et al[8] report improvement of visual scanning with verbal cuing using computer mediated tasks. These gains also generalized to a degree to reading and dialing a telephone. These same authors also report improvement in other visuospatial skills after computer training.

Computer retraining has also been effective with the remediation of visual neglect.[8,19] Some authors caution however, that although there have been indications that computers can assist in the rehabilitation of visual neglect, there is no conclusive evidence that computerized therapy is better than a non-computerized approach.[1,8]

Computer based cognitive retraining has focused primarily on the areas of attention and memory.[20] In a study of 40 head-injured patients who received computer assisted cognitive retraining, significant gains in memory, problem solving and attention were reported.[9] Marks et al[21] report head injury patients who received computer memory retraining improved their memory test performance and that these gains were maintained over time. There was no indication however, if these gains generalized to other tasks. Gilsky[7] reports that T.B.I. patients with memory and learning deficits are able to learn considerable amounts of new knowledge and skills, though at a slower rate than normal, that are relevant to activities of daily living. These goals were accomplished primarily by computer retraining. Training involved the vanishing cues method for which the patient is provided as many initial letters of a target word as needed in order to produce the answer. The computer gradually withdraws the letters across learning trials until the patient is able to answer without cues. He goes on to state that although these goals could be accomplished by other means, the patients in his study tended to like using the computer over other external aids. However, Batchelor et al[14] question these results when reporting the results of their study of forty-seven T.B.I. patients. These authors compared performance of those patients who received computer cognitive retraining with those who received traditional treatment. Their study failed to support the hypothesis that computer training is more effective than traditional treatment in improving memory, attention, information processing and higher cortical functions. In addition, they point out that those studies which claim that computer retraining is better are primarily anecdotal in nature or single case studies.

Increased attentional abilities has also been reported with computer retraining.[18,20] Research has supported the use of the computer as an enhancement to traditional rehabilitation techniques for rehabilitation of attentional deficits. In fact, it is felt that although more research is indicated in order to clarify the mechanisms involved, the research to date suggests that the remediation of attentional skills may be one of the more promising areas of computerized cognitive rehabilitation.[1]

Equally promising is the use of the computer as an adaptive or prosthetic device. One study showed significantly more effective performance on a cooking task with computer generated cuing than without it.[10,11] Another study described a microcomputer organizer which was effective in compensating for the patients decreased memory by increasing functional performance.[22] It is becoming accepted that the microcomputer can be helpful as a memory prosthesis to assist in storage and retrieval of A.D.L. information.[1] Although computer cognitive remediation with the goal of deficit reduction remains controversial, research suggests its use as a cognitive prosthesis is more effective.[12]

Before leaving the topic of computer use in visual, perceptual and cognitive retraining, it is important to address the need for a conceptual framework for its application. Aptly stated by Dunn, The vast array of software being utilized underscores the need for an integrative conceptual framework to guide computer cognitive rehabilitation efforts and allow for the categorization of software in terms of specific cognitive functions.[1] As with any approach, there needs to be a theoretical model or models to guide technology use in rehabilitation and subsequent empirical research which evaluates these efforts.

Several authors recently have attempted to answer this need for a conceptual framework for technology use. Levin[23] outlines six areas of computer use and relates them back to behavioral theory. These six areas are:

1. Computer as a Learning Lab: Client received training in the use of disc drive, mouse etc. Client practices logic and organizational skills within the practical context of applying computer technology.

2. Information Acquisition: Enables experts in particular professional disciplines to create computer assisted resources that imitate their own decision making processes and professional judgment.[23]

3. Computer as Orthotic Device: Simplifies otherwise complex tasks, ex., memory prompts, checklists.

4. Simulations: ie, videogames, practice complex skills in a protected environment.

5. Drill & Practice: Discrete tasks are presented one at a time.

6. Computer Assisted Multitasking: This approach is based on behavioral theory. The emphasis is based on creating ways to help the therapist control environmental contingencies for specific training objectives and goals.

Levin[23] views behavior, including self-managed behavior as based or selected by the environment rather than internal cognitive sources. His computer work is based on this assumption. The therapist arranges training in a hierarchy based on observations of client interaction with the external environment.

Dunn[1] utilizes this concept of the importance of human-environment interactions in his computer work. Dunn conceptualizes a human-machine systems model whereby technology is conceptualized as a highly complex mechanized part of the environment.[1] Interactions between the individual and the computer, or any technology, is a process of input, output and feedback. This human-machine systems model contains two important concepts outlined as follows:[1]

1. Machine assisted approach: Involves temporary use of technology to reduce impairments which lead to disability. For example, training related to attentional deficits.

2. Machine dependent approach: Involves relatively permanent application of technology to accommodate impairment. For example, a speech synthesizer.

In other words, the machine assisted approach is a remedial approach, and the machine dependent an adaptive approach.

In summary, the use of the computer for the rehabilitation of visual, perceptual and cognitive deficits, although retaining continued popularity, remains controversial. Much research justifying its use has lacked adequate control as well as a conceptual base or framework guiding its use. Despite controversy, it is almost universally accepted that the computer is a tool which can be utilized within the context of the intervention method, ie, remedial or adaptive. The effective use of rehabilitation technology requires not just the hardware and software but the "orgware" or human system for appropriate use.[1] In utilizing the computer, the person environment fit must be considered. Future research should contain efficacy studies based on a sound conceptual framework with good controls. Only then, can practice be refined.

References

1. Dunn KW. Information technology and brain injury rehabilitation. In: Finlayson MAJ, Garner SH (eds). *Brain Injury Rehabilitation: Clinical Considerations*. Baltimore, Williams and Wilkins; 1994.

2. Bracy O. Computer based cognitive rehabilitation. *Cognit Rehab.* 1983;1(1):7-8.
3. Hansen CS. Traumatic brain injury. In: Van Deusen J. (ed.) *Body Image and Perceptual Dysfunction in Adults.* Philadelphia: WB Saunders; 1993.
4. Milner D. Use of microcomputers in the treatment of patients with physical disabilities. *Phys Disab Snter Sect Newsletter.* 1984;7(2):1.
5. Weber MP. About this issue. *Phys Disab Spec Inter Sect Newsletter.* 1984;2(2):1.
6. Adamovich BLB. Cognition, language, attention and information processing following closed head injury. In: Kreutzer JS, Wehman PH. (eds.) *Cognitive Rehabilitation For Persons with Traumatic Brain Injury: A Functional Approach.* Baltimore: Paul H. Brooks Publishing Co.; 1991.
7. Glisky EL. Computer-assisted instruction for patients with traumatic brain injury: teaching of domain-specific knowledge. *J Head Trauma Rehabil.* 1992;7(3):1-12.
8. Robertson I, Gray J, Mckenzie S. Microcomputer based cognitive rehabilitation of visual neglect: three multiple baseline single case studies. *Brain Injury.* 1988;2(2):151-163.
9. Ruff RM, Baserr CA, Johnston JW, Marshal LF, Klauber SK, Klauber MR, Minteer M. Neuropsychological rehabilitation: an experimental study with head injured patients. *J.H.T.R.* 1989;4(3):20-36.
10. Kirsch NL, Levine SP, Fallon-Krueger M, Jaros LA. The microcomputer as an "orthotic" device for patients with cognitive deficits. *Journal of Head Trauma Rehabilitation.* 1987;2(4):77-86.
11. Kirsch NL, Levine SP, Lajiness-O'Neill R, Schnyder M. Computer-assisted interactive task guidance: facilitating the performance of a simulated vocational task. *J Head Trauma Rehabil.* 1992;7(3):13-25.
12. Lynch WJ. Software update. *J Head Trauma Rehabil.* 1994;9(2):105-108.
13. Gianutsos R. The computer in cognitive rehabilitation: it's not just a tool anymore. *J Head Trauma Rehabil.* 1992;7(3):26-35.
14. Batchelor J, Shores EA, Marosszeky JE, Sandanam J, Lovarini M. Focus on clinical research: cognitive rehabilitation of severely closed-head-injured patients using computer-assisted and noncomputerized treatment techniques. *J Head Trauma Rehabil.* 1988;3(3):78-85.
15. Lynch WJ. The use of electronic games in cognitive rehabilitation. In: Trexler LE. (ed.) *Cognitive Rehabilitation—Conceptualization and Intervention.* New York: Plenum Press; 1982.
16. Parente R. Cognitive rehabilitation and the use of computers. Paper presented to Baltimore Adult Communications Disorders Interest Group.
17. Parente R, Anderson JK. Techniques for improving cognitive rehabilitation: teaching organization and encoding skills. *Cognit Rehabil.* 1983:20-22.
18. Sohlberg MM, Mateer CA. *Introduction to Cognitive Rehabilitation: Theory and Practice.* New York, The Guilford Press; 1989.
19. Robertson SL, Jones LA. Tactile sensory impairments and prehensile function in subjects with left hemisphere cerebral lesions. *Arch Phys Med Rehabil.* 1994;75:1108-1117.
20. Thomas-Stonell N, Johnson P, Schuller R, Jutai J. Evaluation of a computer-based program for remediation of cognitive-communication skills. *J Head Trauma Rehabil.* 1994;9(4):25-37.
21. Marks C, Parente R, Anderson J. Retention of gains in outpatient cognitive rehabilitation therapy. *Cogn Rehabilitation.* 1986;4(3):20-23.
22. Giles G, Shore M. The effectiveness of an electronic memory aid for a memory-impaired adult of normal intelligence. *Am J Occup Ther.* 1989;43(6):409-411.
23. Levin W. Computer applications in cognitive rehabilitation, In: Kreutzer JS, Wehman PH. (eds.). *Cognitive Rehabilitation for Persons with Traumatic Brain Injury: A Functional Approach.* Baltimore: Paul H. Brooks Co.; 1991.

Additional Current and Related Evaluations Developed by Occupational Therapists

THE ARNADOTTER O.T.-ADL NEUROBEHAVIORAL EVALUATION (A-ONE)[1]

Description:
A 30-45 minute evaluation appropriate for use with patients with central nervous system damage. It simultaneously evaluates the patient's ADL status and neurobehavioral impairments. The A-ONE is divided into two parts. The first part utilizes three scales, i.e., functional independence, (FI) specific neurobehavioral impairment scale (SNBS), and the pervasive neurobehavioral impairment scale (PNBS). Part II of the A-ONE is optional and serves to assist the therapist in localizing lesion site related to exhibited neurobehavioral deficits.

Reliability/Validity:
Extensive reliability and validity measures were performed and are described in: Arnadotter, G. *The Brain and Behavior: Assessing Cortical Dysfunction Through Activities of Daily Living.* St. Louis, C.V. Mosby Co., 1990.
Author's note: This test has great potential for use by occupational therapists because it identifies specific neurobehavioral deficits and how they are interfering with functional independence.

THE RABIDEAU KITCHEN EVALUATION REVISED (RKE-R)[2]

Description:
An assessment of meal preparation skills for adults with traumatic brain injury. It requires the patient to prepare a cold sandwich with two fillings and a hot instant beverage. The evaluation is broken down into 40 component steps which are each scored individually with a three-point scale.

Validity:
Content and criterion related validity were established.

Reliability:
Inter-rater and test-retest were established. Preliminary norms were also generated. Refer to reference #2 for detailed information.

Author's note: This evaluation, with continued reliability and validity research has potential for a comprehensive meal preparation evaluation. It does not at the present time, however, supply the specific reason why the patient is unable to perform a specific component task of the evaluation. Qualitative analysis such as this would greatly enhance its value as an O.T. assessment tool.

References

1. Arnadotter G. *The Brain and Behavior: Assessing Cortical Dysfunction through Activities of Daily Living*. St. Louis, CV Mosby; 1990.
2. Neistadt ME. The Rabideau kitchen evaluation, revised: An assessment of meal preparation skill. *Occup Ther J Research*. Jul/Aug 1992;12(4):242-255.

Evaluation Index

Index